"This is the book I've been pining for. As queer people, we're often left to navigate life and ageing without a map, but Dr Taylor-Pitt has emerged as a wise cartographer who is never afraid to reveal his own vulnerabilities. There is no one way of being queer and no one way of ageing, but Paul has given us all a hell of an atlas."

JOSEPH GALLIANO-DOIG MBE, CO-FOUNDER, QUEER BRITAIN

"Growing up, I thought I was the only boy like me. Growing older, I began to feel alone again – where were the other men like me? Paul's book helped reconnect me to my queerness and engage meaningfully and joyfully with my growing queer community."

DAMIAN BARR, AUTHOR OF *YOU WILL BE SAFE HERE* AND *THE TWO ROBERTS*

"In a world rarely designed with queer people in mind, what a joy to find this smart, thoughtful book."

LAYLA MCCAY, AUTHOR OF *THE QUEER BOOKSHELF* AND *BREAKING THE RAINBOW CEILING*

"Paul gives us permission in his book. Permission to live by our own rules, that we can get it wrong and try again, to reconnect with joy, to love ourselves unconditionally. We have survived dark times and good ones. We absolutely are still here, still queer and ready to live with purpose, unapologetically."

SABA ALI FRSA, EQUALITIES ADVOCATE AND CRITICAL FRIEND

"I came to this book expecting a glimpse of the road ahead; instead, I found a mirror. Warm, funny and fiercely life-affirming, *Still Here! Still Queer! Now What?* honours the histories that made us while offering compassionate, practical ways to become more wholly ourselves. Paul Taylor-Pitt makes ageing feel not like a narrowing of possibility, but an invitation to live more vividly, more deliberately and more queerly. I finished it feeling connected to the generations ahead of me – and excited to join them."

SETH INSUA, AUTHOR OF *HUMAN, ANIMAL* AND *MAN AND WIFE*

"Generation X queer people grew up believing we'd be lucky just to survive, if we even believed we'd survive at all. AIDS shaped our dark, twisted sense of humour (no regrets), our resilience, our relationships and the baggage many of us are only now beginning to unpack. This book is a funny, compassionate and much-needed reminder that surviving was never meant to be the end of our story."

PEACHES CHRIST, FILMMAKER, CULT LEADER

Still Here! Still Queer!
Now What?

of related interest

The Queer Guide to Nutrition and Lifestyle
Daniel O'Shaughnessy
ISBN 978 1 39983 210 6
eISBN 978 1 39983 211 3

Queer Minds
LGBTQ+ Therapists and Advocates on Mental Health, Neurodivergence, and the Things That Help
Katy Lees
ISBN 978 1 80501 181 1
eISBN 978 1 80501 182 8

The Queer Mental Health Workbook
A Creative Self-Help Guide Using CBT, CFT and DBT
Dr Brendan J Dunlop
ISBN 978 1 83997 107 5
eISBN 978 1 83997 108 2

Do You Believe in Life After Loss?
Queer Stories of Loss, Hope and Resilience
Andrew Flewitt
ISBN 978 1 80501 770 7
eISBN 978 1 80501 771 4

STILL HERE! STILL QUEER! NOW WHAT?

A Guide to LGBTQ+ Wellness and Wholeness in Midlife

DR PAUL TAYLOR-PITT

Foreword by Timothy Spoor

Illustrated by Anders Tallvik

Jessica Kingsley Publishers
London and Philadelphia

First published in Great Britain in 2027 by Jessica Kingsley Publishers
An imprint of John Murray Publishing Group

1

A CIP catalogue record for this title is available from the
British Library and the Library of Congress

ISBN 978 1 39984 029 3
eISBN 978 1 39984 030 9
Audio ISBN 978 1 39984 189 4

Printed and bound in Great Britain by Bell & Bain Limited

Jessica Kingsley Publishers' policy is to use papers that are natural, renewable and recyclable products and made from wood grown in sustainable forests. The logging and manufacturing processes are expected to conform to the environmental regulations of the country of origin.

Jessica Kingsley Publishers
Carmelite House
50 Victoria Embankment
London EC4Y 0DZ

www.jkp.com

John Murray Publishing Group
Part of Hodder & Stoughton Ltd
An Hachette Company

The authorised representative in the EEA is Hachette Ireland,
8 Castlecourt Centre, Dublin 15, D15 XTP3, Ireland (email: info@hbgi.ie)

Contents

Part III: Now What?

Resources

For Dan. My nerf herder.

To all those who did not make it this far. Rest in power.

> "There is a vitality, a life force, a quickening that is translated through you into action, and there is only one of you in all time. This expression is unique, and if you block it, it will never exist through any other medium; and be lost. The world will not have it. It is not your business to determine how good it is, nor how it compares with other expressions. It is your business to keep it yours clearly and directly, to keep the channel open. You do not even have to believe in yourself or your work. You have to keep open and aware directly to the urges that motivate you. Keep the channel open. No artist is pleased. There is no satisfaction whatever at any time. There is only a queer, divine dissatisfaction, a blessed unrest that keeps us marching and makes us more alive than the others."
>
> MARTHA GRAHAM

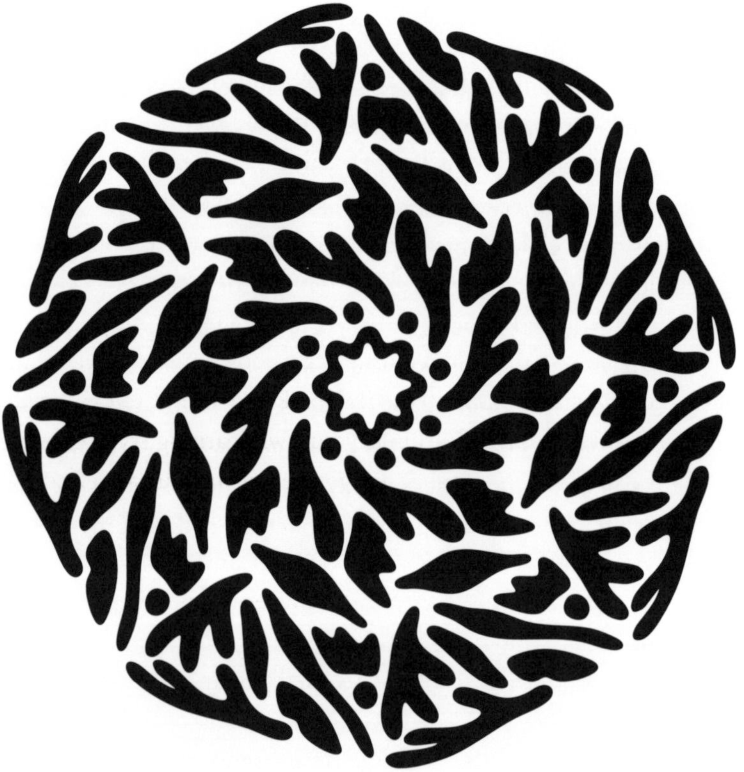

Foreword

As a social worker, charity leader and executive coach who has spent 30 years supporting LGBTQ+ people toward authenticity and self-leadership, I am always searching for works that go beyond platitudes and truly resonate with the complexity of human experience. *Still Here! Still Queer! Now What?* is one such book – a refreshing, heartfelt and empowering companion for anyone navigating the lifelong journey of self-acceptance and belonging.

Structured as a three-part journey, this book is more than a guide, it is a coaching experience. Paul Taylor-Pitt does not tell you what to do. He invites you to lean into your own learning style, offering exercises and techniques that are gentle yet profoundly effective. What struck me most is the way he balances the deeply personal with the collective: while you feel he is speaking directly to you, there is a constant reminder that our power is magnified when we stand together as a community.

This is not another "self-help" manual, it is an act of affirmation. It celebrates who we are, encouraging us to rediscover joy, embrace resilience without guilt, and validate ourselves with compassion rather than chasing external approval. Paul also speaks to the reality that resilience, while essential, can be exhausting, and he meets that truth with honesty and kindness.

I was moved by the book's recognition of the unique challenges faced by midlife folk, the first fully "out" generation. The acknowledgement that coming out, whether to ourselves or others, does not automatically deliver belonging is refreshingly honest. Yet, woven throughout is a powerful reminder: the past, with all its pain and triumphs, pales in comparison to the vast opportunity that lies ahead if we choose to embrace it.

At times, this journey may feel challenging, even uncomfortable, but that is the nature of transformation. The gift of this book is that you never feel alone in that discomfort; you are supported, encouraged and inspired.

Having spent more than 40 years living openly as a queer person and working alongside LGBTQ+ individuals, I found myself both affirmed and re-energized by this book. It is a mirror, a guide and a celebration. Above all, it is a call to step forward into a future rich with possibility.

Still Here! Still Queer! Now What? is a powerful invitation to reclaim your wholeness, courage and joy.

TIM SPOOR FRSA MBE
CHIEF EXECUTIVE, QUEERWELL
QUEERWELL.ORG.UK

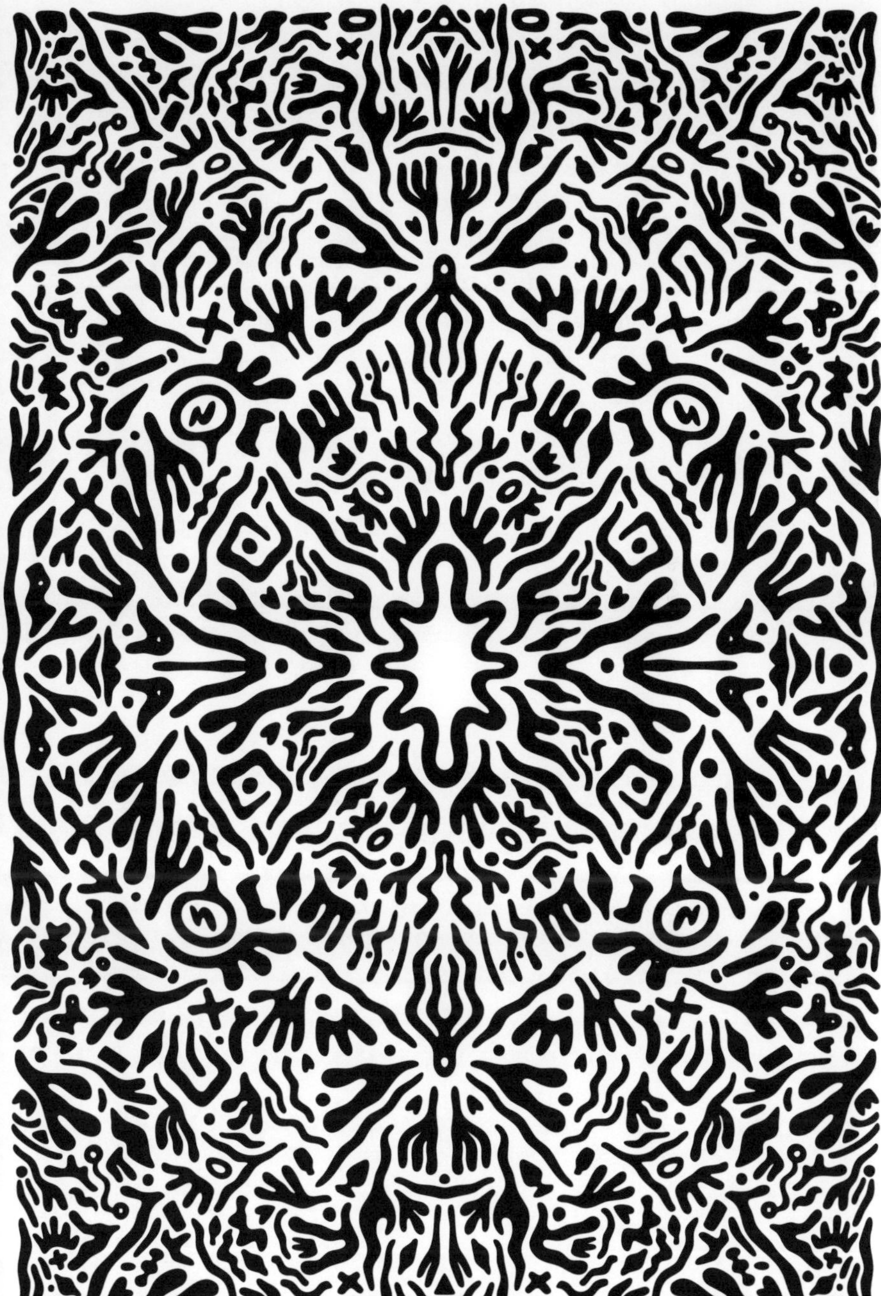

GETTING STARTED

It Took a Village

> "We are a lost generation of LGBTQ+ people. We lost so many before us. Those coming up now have different kinds of friendship networks that we never had growing up. We have very different lived experiences from anyone else alive because of the generation that we grew up in. So, it's definitely an interesting time. I think it's making us all feel a bit lost, like we are floundering sometimes."
>
> – GARETH, 46

In researching this book, I've been told time and again that we just don't talk about the stories of queerness and ageing enough, with all the joys and challenges that happen along the way. Telling these stories is vital, after all. Through sharing our experiences without judgement or embarrassment, having another human being hear them who can empathize with our tales, receiving a gentle nod that says they understand us, we can take off the suits of armour many of us have been wearing for such a long time. It is only then that we can begin to make sense of ourselves, together.

As the cultural context around us has changed and spaces became safer to enter, we – or at least, I know this to be true for myself – may have become complacent. In my case, with that complacency came a gradual, creeping hetero-normification of my life, a beige-washing of my pinkness. I was one of the nice gays next door. I had a good job. A Mini Cooper. We got married. We decorated the outside of the house at Halloween. We were nice, normal neighbours ... until I woke up and realized everything I had fought for and campaigned against was being wasted in this ordinary, easy life. By 40, I was feeling drawn back to Soho (London's most well-known LGBTQ+ neighbourhood, for those outside of the UK) for the first time in decades.

Around 2008, I discovered social media and found it to be the most amazing, friendly place. (Showing my age here!) People like me were exploring new spaces to connect that had never been available before. Facebook exploded, and pokes were exchanged. Then, Twitter took it to a new level of personal interaction, and over the next few years, I started to find my people. Queer people. Everyone was, in general, nice to each other. We invented "tweet-ups" and took our virtual connections into physical spaces. I realized for the first time that creating this kind of social, connected community was possible without having to go to pubs or clubs and risk talking to people who didn't ask to be approached. Social media was incredibly sociable. It helped me reconnect to my queerness and woke me up from suburban slumber with a sharp slap on the bum.

As I approached 50, I knew I could never again allow myself to be just like everyone else. I made a promise to myself, a midlife manifesto, to live vividly, in pursuit of freedom and pleasure, in the queerest way possible from that moment on. That is where the idea for this book was born.

In describing the purpose behind *Still Here! Still Queer! Now What?*, I've often been met – mostly by straight people, but sometimes not – with the question "But why is this needed when everything is equal now?"– which is like a pink rag to this bull. I say "pink" here because I try to smile compassionately with my head slightly tilted, rather than just going in for the kill like I would with a red rag. I try to explain that, yes, things are so much better and, of course, my life is so much easier than those who came before me. I also describe how, after being with my husband for quarter of a century, I am almost paralysed with fear at the thought of losing him. I explain that one of my other fears is that my health declines and I have to move into a care home, where most of the staff and residents are straight. I tell them I would rather be dead than have to go back into the closet as a pensioner. I talk about the ease with which I diminish my achievements and give other people the credit. I describe my tendency to assume that a straight man will find it repulsive if he thought I fancied him. I give examples of how growing up, I heard again and again that people like me ended up sad and lonely, or we were partying all the time and being promiscuous, which came with its own punishment. I explain how becoming sexually active during the height of the AIDS crisis means I still find it difficult to really enjoy sex. I talk about how nobody ever mentioned gay sex when I was growing up except in the same sentences as words like "disease" and "death". I say how wonderful it would have been if anyone, anywhere, had ever told me that sex with another man could be fun instead of fearful. Those are some of the reasons why this book is needed. To clear our souls of the cobwebs that threaten to hang over our latter years.

Still Here! Still Queer! Now What? is a declaration of power for the LGBTQ+ community that celebrates who we are, even when the world does not agree with us. It helps us remember, rediscover and reclaim our power, joy and magic so we may live our most vibrant and vivid expressions of ourselves in a more deliberate way as we emerge into elderhood. The book offers a set of practical and reflective techniques for connecting us to our queer wholeness, blending techniques from coaching, psychology, philosophy, art, culture and queer magic to create a practical way to reconnect to ourselves and each other. The experiences in the book encourage us to move from midlife crisis to queer midlife confidence, navigating life's transitions with compassion and grace.

This book is a portrait of courage, resilience and authenticity. It is a love letter to those who helped us live more truthfully. It is a tribute to the first generation of people who have been able to live openly, legally, fully and wholly ourselves, despite exclusion, misunderstanding and rejection. Above all, the book is a call to action and invitation for us to remember and reclaim the power and wholeness that have always been inside us. It is a promise of hope that we might find ways to thrive into our elderhood.

Middle-aged queers deserve attention. To be put in the foreground. It has been a long time coming. This is the first work of its kind, and while it can never be everything to everyone, it is a start. It is the beginning of a conversation, not the end. I offer this work proudly to queer folk, with love. There is so much we need to do, because despite living in a world that does not care for or want us, we continue to strive for an authentic life.

This is not just a book, it is a celebration that we are still here, still queer and have the chance to live with renewed purpose and pride.

CONVERSATIONS ABOUT QUEERNESS

Alongside my own story, you'll find the experiences of lesbians, gay men, bisexual men and women, pansexuals, trans and non-binary people, gender non-conforming and asexual folk. The queerest of the queer.[1] Along with their queer identities, the voices you will hear come from people of colour, disabled people, neuro-spicy folk, drag queens, artists, accountants, software engineers, death doulas, authors, musicians, actors, Africans, Americans, Australians, Brits, Brazilians and so on. This is a book of diverse experiences. It has to be. As a white, cis-gendered, able-bodied man, this cannot just be my voice. I hope those who contributed so beautifully can see and hear themselves vividly reflected in the work. I will be forever grateful that they gave so much of themselves to shape my thinking for this book.

Although people from all walks of life have contributed to this

1 Many people generously and warmly shared their stories with me in the early stages of researching this work. They don't all define themselves as queer; in fact, some said they hate the word, so I tried my best to explain why I am using it without persuading anyone to accept it. More on that later.

book, one unifying factor among us is our age. We are, generally, between 40 and 60, which is the traditional definition of middle-aged. At the time of writing, that's people born in the late 1960s to early 1980s, also known as Generation X. I know first-hand how hard it was to grow up in that time as a queer person. I hope that the experiences of our generation are never repeated, but there are patterns emerging. The progress I have seen happen in my lifetime so far has been seismic, but it is not as linear as I thought it would be. The pendulum is swinging back hard and for some it barely moved in the first place, so I hold a sense of humility and gratitude for the life I am able to live. I walk the tightrope of hope and rage on a daily, sometimes moment-to-moment basis. I am unapologetic in the fierceness with which I defend the right of our generation to be both optimistic and furious.

Through the process of writing this book, which meant gathering stories from middle-aged queer people, I recognize those feelings – and so many more – in them, too. While everyone is different, middle-aged queers have a lot in common. Who are we? Below are some key similarities that our stories have revealed.

Diversity of identity and background are our strengths

The voices you will read in this book encompass a wide range of identities existing at the same time. There are all flavours of gender, sexuality, race and cultural background. Intersectional identities are woven beautifully through these stories: queer and Black, queer and neurodivergent, queer and closeted – the list goes on. The spectrum of difference is something to be applauded for the richness it brings.

Midlife queers have so much experience to share

Every story I've shared in this book falls into the category of middle-aged, including those at the boundaries of the category. They reflect the unique challenges that come from being at this stage of life, having lived through decades of societal change. We survived the height of the AIDS crisis, when so many did not. We have seen LGBTQ+

rights shift at significant pace. Our narratives are informed by a deep knowing of the historical context in which we exist.

Resilience and adaptability run through our veins

One of the most striking traits that shone through the conversations I had is resilience. So many of the stories I witnessed contained trauma, hardship, rejection, discrimination and personal loss. Despite these challenges, and often because of them, people adapted and found ways to live authentically. Even though we live in a world that does not always welcome us, we have, on the whole, found and claimed our space with tenacity and courage.

We have high levels of self-awareness and insight

The unexamined life is not worth living, even when it looks like a safe place to be. The conversations that informed this work were so densely packed with insight that can only come from deep personal reflection on the most shadow-heavy, sometimes difficult experiences in our lives. The people who shared their stories did not just recount chronological facts, either; they offered analysis and opinion on their experiences, which allowed us to uncover powerful and impactful meaning.

We want authenticity or nothing

Authenticity in these conversations was prized and pursued with vigour. Many of the interviewees talked about spending decades making sense of their true selves in the face of huge societal pressure to conform to heteronormative expectations. The pursuit of authenticity is an important facet of our stories, along with our refusal to be anything other than truly ourselves.

Our only constant is change

It may be tempting to believe that once we come out and establish ourselves into adulthood, the rest of life is smooth sailing, but consistent across these conversations is the theme of change. Lots of change. Whether it involves changing family dynamics, career shifts, marriage, divorce, illness or just facing our own mortality, we are made up of changes that have impacted our values, priorities and senses of self. Change brings an abundance of challenges, but for many of us it also offers tremendous opportunities for growth and self-acceptance.

We advocate for community despite varying degrees of closeness

Our relationship to the LGBTQ+ community is patchy, changing and complex. Many of us have experienced exclusion from the spaces where we should feel most accepted; but despite these frustrating moments, there is still a desire to foster and deepen connections with people like us. We may not be the party animals we once were, but we crave spaces where we can enter into meaningful and uplifting conversation.

The spectre of our mortality hovers near

Many of us are contemplating more deeply our own mortality and the legacy we want to leave behind – if we want to leave behind anything at all. While the concept of our own death is not one that we necessarily welcome, the increasingly concrete knowledge that our time is limited encourages us to consider how we might live consciously in our middle to later age. Conversations about what might happen if our physical and mental health begin to decline weigh heavily on our minds, alongside a desire to make things better for ourselves as we age into elderhood.

> “You feel increasingly invisible as an older queer person. I like talking about this stage of life because we don't have role models. We lost a generation who would have been our role models.”
>
> – STEVE, 52

Of course, not every middle-aged queer person will see themselves in each aspect of the similarities I described above, or within this book's themes. But these are starting points for a wider and deeper set of conversations, a place for us to build more intelligence and insight by expanding the ways we talk about what it's like to be a middle-aged queer person.

For me, speaking with so many queer people about their experiences was humbling and invigorating. Some of the stories were so similar to my own that I had to interrupt the speaker and ask if they had been reading my journal. Others were so wildly different that they took my breath away. During the conversations, we laughed, cried, shared and sat in silent moments of disbelief or wonder. Many of the people I interviewed told me they had never spoken to anyone about themselves so honestly before. Most had never been asked to.

Not only was it a privilege to witness their stories unfolding before me, but I also felt an increasing sense of power emerging. The energy being absorbed into my brain was electric. I understood a new sense of responsibility for holding these precious tales, while at the same time experiencing a growing restlessness to put them to use and honour them. I worried that I wouldn't be able to do them justice. I still hold some of that fear. To listen and be listened to is one of the most significant gifts we can offer another human. Making something with the knowledge that is created when many stories come together is a blessing I have taken very seriously.

As I said, it did not sit lightly with me that I was often hearing things that had never been spoken aloud before. Equally, I was responding to this openness with a new sense of boldness in how I showed up to the conversations. And, in turn, I also shared stories nobody had ever heard before – some of those stories are in this book. It has been an incredibly powerful process. I felt alive, connected and part of a collective in a way I hadn't experienced before.

I offer my personal stories with a healthy dose of trepidation, and I worry about exposing myself and those close to me to scrutiny that may not be welcomed. The experiences I have brought to life in these pages are curated from a life of complex feelings and thoughts.

Everything I have written about is true, to the extent of my knowing that sometimes I remember an event and other times I believe I remember it because I am looking at a photo of it. While I pride myself to be a reliable narrator of my own life, by the time I reached 50 I had embraced so many catchphrases from *French & Saunders*, Victoria Wood, Jenny Eclair, Sandra Bernhard and Judy Garland that I sometimes mistake their words for my own.

Everything I've shared is offered in good faith, and I hope that it may be responded to in a similar way. This work is deliberately aimed at a segment of the population who need it. The opinions of anyone else are irrelevant. Some people will reject and vilify the need for this book to exist, as they do for us in general. It doesn't matter what they think. No amount of critique or criticism will affect how I feel about myself. It may have taken half a century, but I can stand with my arms outstretched and my heart exposed, knowing that everything that belongs to me can never be diminished by anyone. Like Björk on the cover of her Vulnicura album, my wounds are on show but only because I choose to show them.

It has been said that you write the book you need to read. After writing this book, I utterly believe that. I have had the luxury of reading along as I wrote it, testing out the exercises and seeing myself change and grow through the process. I have first-hand experience of using the material and feeling better about myself. I'm looking forward to *Still Here! Still Queer! Now What?* doing the same for you.

QUESTIONS ABOUT OUR QUEERNESS

> "I'll speak to younger friends and they're like, 'Oh, yeah, I'm gonna have three kids,' or whatever. I just think, How bloody cool is that? It's just a part of everyday gay conversation. It never crossed my mind. No way."
>
> – DOM, 57

It was a privilege to ask questions to the people who volunteered to be part of this book. I asked so many questions, perhaps in an attempt to find answers for myself. I have reached middle age with a nagging question in my mind: *How did I get here?* That's quickly followed by: *And what is "here" like?* I then finally ask myself: *And what the fuck do I want from the rest of my life?*

These are big questions, but thankfully, I'm a huge fan of big questions. I believe the questions we ask ourselves are an amazing way to learn and grow. Questions asked with sincerity are a rope ladder that can save us from drowning, or an invitation to lift our heads toward the stars. So, this book is full of questions. Lots of questions.

I have also included my own answers to those questions as a way of illustrating the process, but they belong to me only and should not be taken as anything other than one person's view on this. My biggest hope is that you'll ask yourself these questions and respond to them – and then ask someone else and hear their answers. As with life, the process is often more interesting than the task. How we get to an answer can be more revealing than the answer itself! But if you do find answers, that is even more delicious.

To get us going on this adventure of ours, I'd like to begin with some questions that might require some deep reflection over a period of days, or you might find that your replies come to you in an instant, like a bolt of lightning. I'd like you to recall, in as much vivid detail as possible ...

- Where you were ...
- What the weather was like ...
- What you were wearing ...
- What you had just eaten ...
- What kind of smells were in the air ...
- What the ground felt like under your feet ...
- What sounds were around you, nearby and in the distance ...
- Who you were hanging around with ...
- What was on TV ...

- What songs were on the radio ...
- What your favourite book was ...
- Who you fancied ...
- What kind of cars were on the road ...
- Who was running the country ...
- What the biggest news story was at the time ...

... when you first came out to yourself.

There's space for your notes here.

Did anything surprise you in your reflection? Think of it as data that we'll be adding to throughout the book.

Now that we are off and running, let's go into a bit more detail on how this book works.

CHASING WHOLENESS

Wholeness is a relatively recent goal for me. During the first Covid-19 lockdown, I started a podcast called *Hopecast* with a wonderfully quirky and diverse group of guys. We met through an online meditation group, and they all said yes when I suggested creating a podcast. The "hope" in *Hopecast* stood for **H**omos **O**f **P**lanet **E**arth, as we were scattered around the world in places like London, Lisbon, Amsterdam and Atlanta. For almost two years and 80 episodes, we talked about sexuality, spirituality, wellness and queerness. In many ways, *Hopecast* is the seed from which this book grew. I took great joy in naming each of the episodes, my favourite of which was called "Glory Whole". It was a deceptively playful title as it encompassed joy, queer sex, wholeness and pleasure in two words.

I became a little obsessed with the idea of wholeness alongside wellness. To me, wellness is a state of being that can be improved by external factors such as food, massage, a comfy bed and a pair of running shoes. Wholeness, on the other hand, is deeper and more introspective. I don't believe anyone else can make me whole. My sense of wholeness is entirely my responsibility. So, I began to explore the idea of queer wholeness, which led me to understand that my – our – queerness is a bone-deep vital element of feeling whole. My queerness has been part of me as long as my first cells. My queerness makes me whole. I realized I had forgotten that over the years as the outside world picked away at it. But in middle age, I felt ready to remember and reconnect to the power of my queer wholeness.

So, this book is written for us, the midlife queer folk. While some of our wholeness may have been fractured, it is still and has always been there waiting to be (re-) discovered. For me there's a huge excitement in that. You might feel it too. In fact, you might be so revved up that you want to dive straight in. I salute you for that. You're the Tom Daley of the reading world, except older and maybe struggling to get into those Speedos, but don't ever let anyone tell you not to try.

You should know that in these pages are stories of victimhood, shame and self-loathing. Conversations about love, loss and lust. Tales of depression, isolation and rejection. These are all deliberately included. It's my equivalent of using one of those foot-grater tools on a rough heel to get to the nice, smooth bit underneath. Sorry for putting that image in your mind. It's important to explore these emotive topics, and they seem to resonate among queer folk of our generation. So, be aware that as you read, you might come across things that feel difficult or challenging. Be sure to be kind and gentle to yourself. At the back of the book is a list of resources and places you might go to if you find yourself getting overwhelmed by some of the themes.

To dip our toes even deeper into the waters of self-reflection, let's consider some more questions that have an optimistic, celebratory feel.

QUESTIONS TO PONDER

What is the best, most brilliant thing about being you?

Where would you love to shine even more brightly?

How might it be to be seen exactly as you wish to be?

How did you find answering those questions? Maybe you found it easy to compliment yourself, or perhaps it felt weird or uncomfortable. Whatever happened is fine and right. Understanding our reactions and responses is such valuable knowledge. That's where this book can help. *Still Here! Still Queer! Now What?* is a toolkit for becoming, feeling and being whole using three new tools: The Queer Wheel of Midlife, The Queer Wholeness Method and The Queer Midlife Manifesto. We can use these tools when we feel a little stuck, confused or lost in those moments when we think about who we've been and who we crave being. The process of using the tools will bring us closer to remembering and being exactly who we are and want to be. To feeling whole.

When we unapologetically stand in the power of our queer wholeness, we change ourselves, each other and the world for good. To begin, let's explore something you'll see throughout the book: the word "queer".

QUEER

WHY QUEER?

> "I've got a tattoo on my wrist; it's a box that is a symbol of the 'Other' checkbox on a form. It's a reminder that it's okay not to fit neatly into the main options and that being 'other' can be useful, even powerful. It's taken me a long time to get to a place where I truly feel that, but I'm finally there."
>
> – LIZI, 40

Vi Taylor, my 97-year-old Aberdonian nana, described people she thought were weird as "affa queer" or, in English, awfully unusual. She used the word "queer" with absolutely no malice at all. It was just a word she had always used as a throwaway term for something like a cat with only three legs, or how she felt after eating a dodgy sandwich.

Words and their meaning are always changing, sometimes slowly and at other times faster than the speed of sound. The word "queer" has been with us for hundreds of years, making its first appearance in the English language during the 16th century. At that time, it was not exactly an insult, but could be used to mean odd, eccentric, peculiar – maybe a descriptor for someone who wore a feather in their hair on Tuesdays.

In the 19th century, queer started to be used in common conversation to refer to men who were attracted to each other. It was not used politely. Despite that, it makes me glow inside to know that in 1873, one hundred years before I was born, men were fucking men and being called queer for it. We have always been here. Around the time of my birth, although not directly related (as far as I know), queer people had taken enough of straight people's bullshit and decided to fight back. They reclaimed queer and stripped it of its hurtful power, chanting, "We're here! We're queer! Get used to it!"

In the 1990s, queer meant more than just being gay. It took on an increasingly political edge, a spirit of rebellion – "not gay as in 'happy', queer as in 'fuck you'" – to challenge the restrictive and heteronormative expectations placed on us by society. In 1992, Australian soap star Jason Donovan sued The Face magazine for publishing a faked photo of him wearing a t-shirt that said "queer as fuck". His libel case was successful. He was awarded £292,000 in damages for the slur of being called queer.

In the 21st century, queer has come to be an inclusive term used by anyone who doesn't identify as heterosexual or cisgender, for those who don't feel words like "gay", "lesbian" or "bisexual" are the best fit for them, and encompasses all the beautiful fluidity of gender and sexual identity. Queer remains proudly political.

Around the world, queer can be translated into some other languages, but it is rarely direct and depends a lot on the cultural context. In Spanish, queer can be translated to *cuir* – pronounced the same – where it retains most of its meaning. The French translation *estrange* literally means strange. In Germany, they have a word to specifically describe gay men – *schwul* – whereas in Japan, there is no word for queer. Language has the power to embrace or exclude. Queer not being understood everywhere shows that the world has not yet come to terms with our existence.

Queer still causes reactions. While it has been reclaimed from an insult to a term of empowerment, and even endearment, it has been for me a useful tool in my own path to self-acceptance. Where once I had the word thrown at me, now I have it proudly tattooed on my chest. And yet, I still have an almost physical response when I see the word unexpectedly. I saw a guy at the gym wearing a t-shirt covered in words like "music", "dance", "party" and "queer". The latter was the first word I noticed. It was on his back. My first thought was, How will he see someone coming up behind him so he can defend himself? Clearly, the word still signals danger to my subconscious. I have work to do on my relationship with it, and maybe even with what it means to be queer.

I used "queer" deliberately in the title of this book and the methods it describes. Rather than calling it "Rainbow Wholeness" or "Gay Wholeness", it felt important to me that I attended to my Queer Wholeness. It means my methods for doing so are applicable to anyone who relates to or identifies with any of the definitions that come under queer's big, comfy arms.

QUESTIONS TO PONDER

What does the word "queer" evoke for you?

When did you first become aware of words describing sexuality?

What is your preferred term for describing your sexuality?

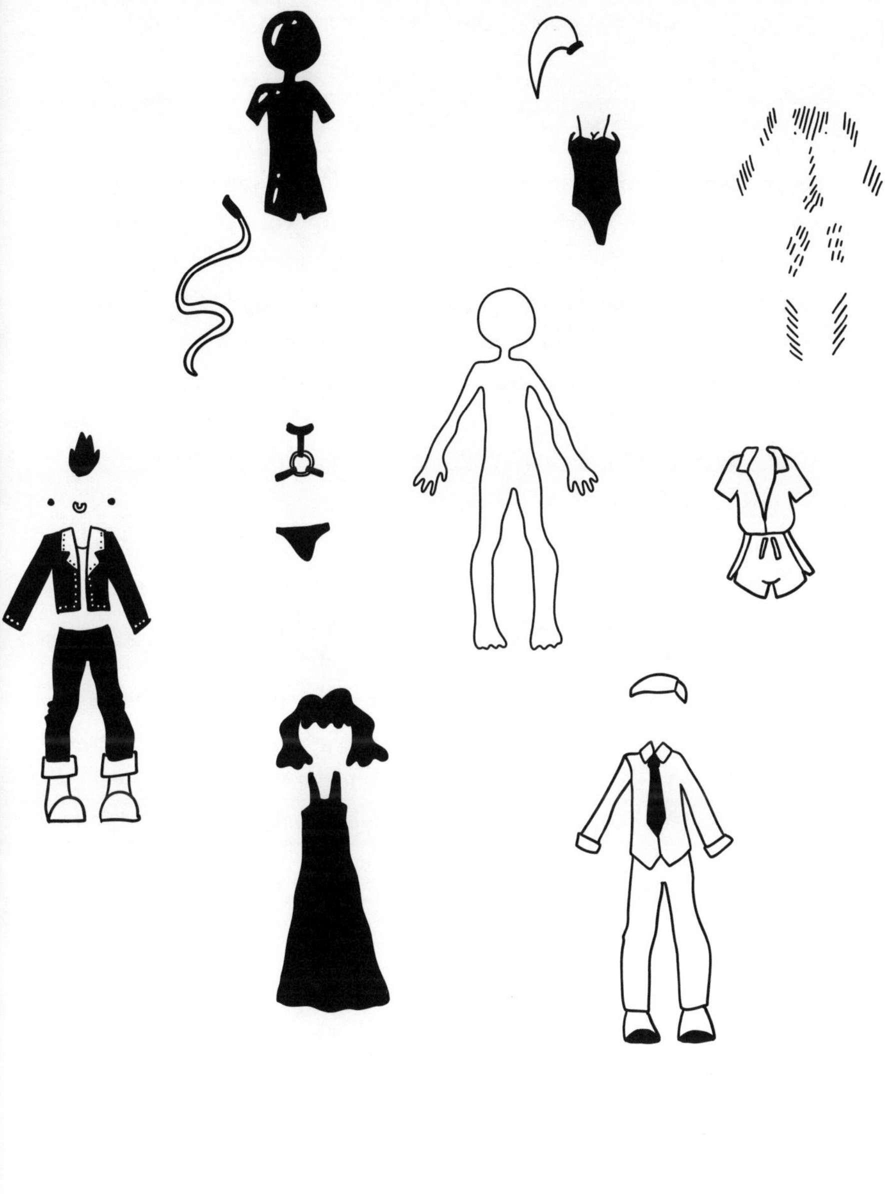

SOMEWHERE BETWEEN GROWING UP AND GETTING OLD

> "I wish I'd had the courage to come out earlier because when you don't, you deny yourself the truth of your existence. You live a half life."
>
> – RAGA, 54

Something called you to pick up this book. Was it the cover? Maybe you liked the title. It could be that you heard a whisper that encouraged you to get it, or perhaps it was a cry from your soul. Only you know the path that led you to have this in your hand today. This is your opportunity to reflect on where you have come from, what it's like to be where you are now and who you might want to be in the future. These are big conversations, but we have run out of time to waste it on small thoughts. We deserve nothing less than everything at this point in our lives.

Middle-aged queer people made it to where we are without much help from the world. The path offered to us took us through terrain we didn't recognize – half-lit roads, sharp bends, fierce climbs – but we made it through. Our stories are those of adventurers, pioneers and travellers who have spanned seismic shifts, feeling cultural tectonic plates move under our feet. We are a generation with experiences that no one had before us, and that no one will ever have again. Our unique tales are rarely shared because our queerness and our age often subject us to a double layer of invisibility. Homonegative, biphobic and transphobic people turn their backs on us if we're lucky, and deliberately try to make our lives awful if we're not. Younger queer people forging their own paths might think we are over the hill and past our usefulness.

And yet, we are still here. Many of us have survived the worst kind of horrors, and others have managed more minor traumas. Some of us made it here unscathed, with only small scratches. Few, if any, of us arrived here in one piece. To be here now may come with a feeling of guilt since so many of our folk did not make it this far. Their voyages were cut short by epidemics, partying or the pressure of an uncaring world. We, however, have the chance to live more deliberately.

What is *here* like? And at this stage of life, are we where we hoped we would be? Maybe we have exceeded the limited expectations of a society that does not wish for us to succeed. Perhaps we have achieved more than we ever believed we could. Some of us might be in an okay place with no major grumbles, while others are simply not where we want to be.

We could not be ourselves for a long time and we might still find it hard to do that now. There may be aspects of our lives that need attention, compassion and care. A few places might feel like they are on fire. All of that is welcome here, and it's always changing.

Consider where you are in your life

Before going any further into these pages, pause for a moment and consider these questions:

- What is this book asking of you?
- Is there a part of you that is seeking change, or growth, or nurturing?
- What would it be like to invite any or all of those parts of yourself to turn up their volume?
- What would these voices say? What would they want for you?

With these voices in mind, encourage one of them to speak up.

- What does it desire for you?
- Where might it like you to pay some attention?

Now, widen your lens.

- If you were to focus on something that might make your life feel like you are living it more deliberately, more authentically, more wholly, what would that be?

- By the time you get to the end of the book, how would you like to feel?
- How would you know if the investment of time, money or energy into this book has been worth it for you?

QUESTIONS TO PONDER

Answer the questions on the previous pages in this space.

A wish for yourself

Finally, what is the wish you want to make for yourself – one that nobody else ever needs to know – that, if you achieved it, would mean you are closer to who, where and how you really want to be?

Make the wish. Say it silently to yourself. Maybe you could be bold and whisper it. Could you consider shouting it? If you feel extra courageous, you could write it down here so that you can come back to it later.

A wish for myself:

HOW TO USE THIS BOOK

> “In Brazil, there are lots of soap operas. In one of them, there was a gay character – he dressed like a woman, a real stereotype. But there was a scene in that soap opera that made him very human, so I thought, I'm going to talk to my father. Well, wow. Yeah, it was hard. He told me that I should look for a priest. Look for a doctor. Look for a psychologist. He didn't accept it."
>
> – EDUARDO, 41

The main body of this book is split into parts which contain methods and models you can follow at your own pace, in your own time. Each part explores elements of our past, present and future queerness.

- STILL HERE! (Part I) is all about knowing yourself. We'll start wherever you are now and spend some time exploring how you got to where you are. It's the foundation for all the work that comes next, building on your insights and knowledge of your own story. This part includes The Queer Wheel of Midlife, a tool you can use to work out where you are in relation to key themes that emerged from the interviews that informed the content of this book. Each theme is accompanied by a short piece of writing that illustrates my own experience with the topic. The Queer Wheel of Midlife will help you work out where you might want to focus some attention and make some changes.

- STILL QUEER! (Part II) introduces The Queer Wholeness Method, an interactive set of exercises and experiments to help you more fully experience your beautiful and powerful queer wholeness. The method aims to guide you in locating and opening your sense of wholeness, with the hope that you may be able to expand it and show it to others more easily and naturally. Wholeness is our hidden superpower, often forgotten when living in a world that seeks to fracture our senses of self. The Queer Wholeness Method uses your brain and body to experience what it might mean to be even more whole.

- NOW WHAT? (Part III) invites you to consider The Queer Midlife Manifesto, where we turn our insights and learning into practical, positive steps for how we might more deliberately live the lives we want. The Queer Midlife Manifesto is a celebration of the power of our queerness and explores how it can propel us toward an even better and more beautiful way of being. Creating a Queer Midlife Manifesto gives us a vocabulary for talking to each other about our hopes and wishes for the next part of our lives.

The final chapter of the book takes the work you've done individually and connects it to community, exploring how we might deepen and broaden our links to other midlife queers at home and around the world.

All of that is to come, but let's start with where you are right now.

PART I

STILL HERE!

> My mum had a week off work when I told her I was gay.
>
> – JAMES, 41

GETTING TO KNOW YOU

> It's strange, because I think when I hit 50 ... it's not a midlife crisis, but you go, like, what am I doing with my life?"
>
> – DARREN, 51

Let's start off with a seemingly simple yet often very challenging question: Who are you?

Knowing ourselves is key to opening up possibilities for change, which is why we're starting with an exploration of how you got to where you are. You might want to spend a bit of time thinking about who you are now and compare it to who you have been. I am not a naturally reflective person – I'm more interested in what comes next than what happened before – but I find it so useful to give myself time to appreciate the shifts in my life from when I grew up until now.

I was a strange little child in some ways. Quiet. Not shy exactly, but thoughtful. I was never rowdy, nor did I cause any trouble. I had no siblings, so I would spend most of the time at home watching TV. *The Adventure Game* was my favourite show when I was a kid. Every episode, three minor celebrities would board a space shuttle to a mysterious planet populated by friendly shape-shifting monsters who got their kicks from setting puzzles for the humans to solve. Each puzzle won them a token they could use in the final test where they crossed a bridge over space, hoping not to be evaporated by a space twister and sent into the vortex. Nobody won anything at the end. No money exchanged hands. They just enjoyed playing the game, hoping they would survive until the end. A lot like life.

In hindsight, my love for *The Adventure Game* reveals everything about who I was as a child. I was nerdy, obsessed with science-fiction and envious of the ability of the monsters to change shape. I loved the idea that people could transform themselves, while remaining true to who they were at heart. On some level, it gave me hope.

I didn't have a terrible childhood, but it wasn't great either. My fascination with characters who could transform or shapeshift spoke to the part of me that wanted to be someone else. I never had a problem with my sexuality, ever. I must have been born with an inbuilt force field that inexplicably repelled homophobia, or at least stopped it from seeping into my soul. I always knew that it was other people who had the problem, not me. It didn't mean I felt comfortable navigating the straight world, but it did protect me from internalizing the poison.

So, our ability to change has always fascinated me. It led me to study psychology and pursue a career where I work with people, teams and organizations who want to reinvent themselves. I find it hugely inspiring to hold space for someone and watch a spark of an idea burst into flames when they get an image of who, how, what or where they want to be. My job is simply to be the air in the room that keeps the flame alight, rather than a cold bucket of water that snuffs it out. Helping others change helps me change.

THE PAST CAN HELP US CHANGE THE PRESENT

When we change as individuals, it's rarely in isolation. Change happens in relationship with – and in relation to – others: partners, lovers, family, friends, community, counsellors, teams, groups. Real transformation can happen in the absence of others, of course, but it is so much easier and more enduring when it takes place in the presence of someone else. When whole groups of people set out to change something, it can be seismic.

Four years before I was born, the Stonewall riots happened in New York in the summer of 1969. Those bitches had fucking had enough. They decided no more and took matters into their own hands. The events that followed, which all happened in my lifetime, are almost too monumental to believe. In the time I have been alive, homosexuality has been decriminalized in my country of birth (Scotland), and is no longer considered a mental disorder. We can marry our partners, be out at work and fight for the country in the armed forces. We can start families of our own, whether through physical, medical or legal means. It's dizzying how much has changed.

Despite all this progress, it is still not okay for all of us everywhere. I am still not okay all the time. Life is good on the whole, but as I navigate middle age, I notice new and different things that preoccupy me. I think more about death, for example. Not in a morbid way, I hope, but more like knowing it's just outside of my peripheral vision. I wonder what the next 10, 20, maybe even 30 years of my life will be and if my physical or mental health is robust enough to carry me into older age. I fear the loss of loved ones more acutely and carry in my heart more names of those already gone with each passing year. Generally, I am fortunate, happy and grateful to be alive. Yet there's a nagging, consistent feeling that some things could be ... different. Better. That I might live more deliberately. It's confusing sometimes.

As a queer 52-year-old, I do get a little overwhelmed by the amount of history through which I'm living. While so much of it has changed things for the better, for the first time in my life I see society going backward. The progress that I once only dreamed of became a reality; now, that same progress feels more precarious. It is deeply unsettling to experience the wave of hostility that has been building over the last decade. For example, social media has transformed from a safe space for queer communities into somewhere we face non-stop abuse from strangers. Transphobia has intensified in painful and prolific ways. Workplace action around Diversity, Equality and Inclusion, which is proven to contribute to improved performance, has come under attack, with faint-hearted employers rolling back their promises as higher profits trump accepting all types of people. I guess there hasn't ever been a time when it is truly simple and easy to live as a queer person, but I thought we were getting there.

Now, I'm finding myself more guarded again, bracing for the impact of the tightening grip of right-wing ideology on a fragile world. It makes me afraid for the future, but I am not helpless in this story. The fear sparks action and a refusal to allow this backward slide to continue. Succumbing to the forces of bigotry is not an option – not then, not now, not ever. We will get through this, even if the days ahead seem darker. I have experienced dark days in the past and can see a brighter future, but the only way to create that is in the present. Writing this book has allowed me to explore my own past, present and future, sharing the process with others who may want to do the same.

AIMING FOR ACCEPTANCE AND ADAPTABILITY

This book is full of contradictions. It is about radical, unconditional self-acceptance, and it is also about life-altering transformational change. It helps us realize that we are all perfect exactly as we are, and also that we have the potential to change any aspect of ourselves that we want to. This book will help you accept yourself and change yourself. It is not a book about loving yourself. Sometimes liking myself is difficult, never mind loving myself. Feelings and emotions about ourselves are complex, irrational and very personal. They are entirely subjective. My idea of loving myself might be very different to yours, and that is absolutely fine.

Where I believe we may agree is that acceptance and change are vehicles to get to know ourselves better and be more kind to whatever feelings about ourselves we might be with at any particular moment in the day. I want you to accept yourself and change yourself, in whatever ways you like, as I will too.

IN THIS TOGETHER

Growing up, I had very few, if any, positive role models. These days, I learn so much from young folk. They are great at shaping the collective direction of progress, but they can't teach me how to live the rest of my life. They do not have my experiences, for better or worse. As I seek to understand my past, examine the present and imagine the future, I wonder more and more how to live the second half of my life with deeper connections. I want to change myself, inspire myself, and generally to be better. Do better. Feel better.

If that sounds daunting to you, because it certainly does to me, I offer you a hand and the invitation to do it together. I don't think I can do this on my own, but knowing that others might be treading similar paths gives me the courage and strength to keep going.

In some ways, it would be easier to just get on with it and place my head in the sand. Awful, but easier. Examining our more shadowy parts is not always pleasant work. I encounter resistance whenever I bump up against a limiting belief that I hold about myself because at some time, that belief kept me safe. It takes guts to power through, let it go and rewrite some of these old narratives that no longer serve us. So, shall we do it together?

Ultimately, this work in finding ourselves and figuring out who we are comes from a place of joy. Too much has been said about us that no longer serves us, if it ever even did. This applies most of all to those of us in the space of middle age, who grew up in a time of rapid societal shifts. We felt the tide turn and we rode the wave, watching laws change and attitudes bend in a positive direction. Things got so much better for so many of us. Where we are now is in a state of flux. The gains we made are being consistently and deliberately chipped away, eroded by an increasingly toxic tone of voice used in conversations about queerness. That toxicity has always been there. For a while, it seemed like we were winning the battle, and the concentration of toxicity had diluted. Some of it may even have been washed away. Now, though, that toxicity seems to be back with emboldened strength.

It might be easy – and even lazy – to believe that young people are the answer. Maybe they are. It's certainly a lot more common and even acceptable for kids at school to be open about their queerness and live their lives with authenticity. It's also true that they are being taught by people far less cool than they are.

I believe that we, *all of us*, are the future. We are all responsible for leading ourselves, and some of us extend that to leading others. There's both a power and sadness that comes with that. On the one hand, how liberating is it to know that nobody else needs to be concerned with my life other than me? The sadness comes when so many believe they have the right to comment on, judge, legislate and have authority over how we as queer people can live our lives. We are the only people who can do something about that. Straight people are not coming to save us. We are all we have. Are we enough?

TAKING STOCK

So many of us who have reached middle age still don't believe that we are enough. We grew up listening to stories told about us that were not true, and sometimes we believed them anyway. Our queerness did not have the same opportunity to breathe and thrive as it might have if we were young today. All around us, the images of ourselves that we saw were distorted into unrecognizable cliches, twisted monsters and broken victims. If we saw ourselves represented in popular culture, it was often better to look away. Politicians debated our right to live and love legally. The rights enjoyed by the majority were often denied to us altogether, or otherwise served to us as crumbs that we were told we should be grateful for. We grew up in a world that did not want us to exist. We can't not be affected by that. So far, so depressing. Isn't this book supposed to come from a place of joy?

At the heart of my wisdom, if indeed I have gained any in the years leading to middle age, is a belief that change is indeed possible, despite – or maybe because of – what we have been through in the past.

The things that happened to us – good and bad and everything in between – are done. Over. History. They may still show up in our present, as shadows or beacons, signals or stories, but they are only ever an echo. What's done is done. Joy comes from an understanding that we have some power and control over what happens to us in the present which, in turn, creates our futures. The choices we make today shape tomorrow, and there's an abundance of joy in knowing that. In middle age, we can take stock of where we are, how we got here and what might happen next for us. There are many gifts that come with ageing. One is perspective.

In midlife, we can step back, half-close our eyes and look at where we are with a bit more detachment. We can understand how some of the things that we went through led to the choices that we made which, in turn, brought us to this time and place. We get to see our lives as they are and imagine what they could be like as we move forward. Despite all the damage inflicted on us, we are still here. We are still queer. We get to choose what happens next and who we will be throughout it all.

This book is an opportunity to think more deliberately about the rest of your life. You are about to go on the adventure of your lifetime, a journey into wholeness. Your queer wholeness. It's a place where you can be utterly yourself with no need for approval or acceptance from anyone. The path to queer wholeness leads to a place where you can remember and reclaim the power of who you are.

QUESTIONS TO PONDER

What do you already know about yourself?

. . . .

. . . .

. . . .

. . . .

What is characteristic of you?

. . . .

. . . .

. . . .

. . . .

. . . .

How have you learned this?

. . . .

. . . .

. . . .

. . . .

. . . .

What is being you like?

. . . .

. . . .

. . . .

. . . .

. . . .

QUEER WHOLENESS

“A work colleague once said to me, in total seriousness, ‘You’ll never understand love because you’ve never had a child,’ and I almost lost my shit. It was so condescending and patronizing that I couldn’t possibly know what love is because I haven’t pushed a kid out of my vagina.”

– ROB, 41

As we begin this section, consider: How whole do you feel most days? And what do you make of that? What might be getting in the way of making you feel completely whole?

Wholeness happens at every level of life, from the cellular to the celestial. Wholeness is not just our right – it's built into our operating system from birth. We are born whole. We can live whole. We may even die whole. Wholeness means an internal feeling of completeness, of rightness, of okay-ness. To be whole is to be utterly ourselves in every situation. Wholeness is power. Wholeness is control. Wholeness is giving ourselves permission to hope. Wholeness is understanding we never have to compromise who we are. It is the deepest sense of knowing that we are perfectly capable of being wonderfully ourselves. Wholeness is energy. Wholeness is life. Wholeness is freedom. Wholeness is overcoming sabotage. Wholeness is the ability to exist in a hostile world without fear.

My sense of wholeness varies from day to day. Sometimes I give it no thought at all, and other times it's visible and almost tangible. I do need to be reminded of it regularly, though.

OUR UNDERSTANDING OF WHOLENESS

In researching this book, I was struck by the lack of queer voices on this topic. Straight people talk about it a lot. At first, I set myself a task of only including queer thinkers, but it would have been very difficult, as we have been marginalized from so many spaces, including academia and thought leadership. So, I have graciously included some straight voices in the book on the condition that they behave themselves and don't get all weird.

The physicist and philosopher David Bohm, who was openly straight, spoke of the universe as an "unbroken whole". His work set out to explain the workings of the cosmos, describing how all reality and consciousness are part of an essential, unbroken wholeness. More (straight) thinkers and therapists, from Karl Jung to Fritz Perls to Alain de Botton, affirm the idea of wholeness as central to the enduring unfolding of our potential.

A rare queer voice in the canon of existentialism is Michel

Foucault, whose work on sexuality and power fits nicely into conversations on wholeness. Foucault describes wholeness as an integral part of identity, often shaped by societal views.

I don't know what I believe the essence of the "self" looks like, or even what to call it. The "soul" feels too religious; the "spirit" too esoteric. The self feels more right for me, but I still need to use a bit of imagination to picture what this self of mine looks like. When I close my eyes and dream, it's a bright glow, like Mr Burns in *The X-Files* episode of *The Simpsons*. It brings me peace. It brings me love. It also has a few cracks in it. Luckily, these did not come from the physical hands of anyone else. My cracks are from the words, looks, attitudes and culture that I lived through as I grew up, and still experience today. Despite those cracks, I know that my fuzzy, glowing self is still, remarkably, whole. Wholeness feels accessible to me. It has always been there, and nothing can break it.

BARRIERS TO OUR WHOLENESS

Things do get in the way of wholeness – I need to add some balance here. I'm not saying I've got it figured out, or that I don't have plenty to work on. Take my feelings about perfectionism, for example. I have a weird relationship to failure and imperfection. A few years ago, at the start of my doctorate, I spent a silly amount of money on something from The School of Life, a high-priced self-improvement and mental health brand. It's called the Imperfection Pot. It's a pretty little blue-green jug, deliberately made to be imperfect. To me it looked absolutely correct, but apparently it has imperfections. Its creation was inspired by the Japanese philosophy of wabi-sabi, which celebrates life's beauty and simplicity, as well as its flaws, in both nature and in manufactured creations.

There was a reason for me to buy this expensive pot at the time. I had a miniature meltdown six months into my doctorate, as I had convinced myself of a number of things:

- I was going to fail.
- I knew nothing about the topic.
- I probably shouldn't have been doing the job I was in.
- I shouldn't have attempted a doctorate when I couldn't even pass my master's the first time.
- I was the child of an alcoholic teenage mother who was brought up on a council estate – I was not good enough or worthy enough to succeed at anything.
- I should just give up.

You get the picture. At moments like those, I would bring out the Imperfection Pot and stare at it, trying to absorb the beauty of its imperfect wonderfulness. I would tell myself that it's okay to be imperfect. After a while, I would feel confident enough to press "send" on the assignment that was making me feel so wretched.

A year or so into the doctorate, we moved house – why not, it's just another huge life event – and I forgot about the Imperfection Pot. Three years later, when it came time to start writing my 75,000-word thesis, I was again visited by the ghosts of self-sabotage and decided I should bring the pot back out. I looked for it, casually at first, wondering where it went after the house move. I became more confused when I couldn't find it anywhere, and so in typical procrastination mode, I decided to empty one of the moving boxes that was as still untouched. At the bottom of the box, wrapped in a thick towel, was a small, hard, square shape. I peeled back the towel to see the wooden box of the Imperfection Pot, obscured by a layer of bubble wrap sellotaped tightly to itself. Under the wrap, I felt the familiar contours of the lid and slid it open. Inside, the Imperfection Pot itself was wrapped in newspaper and nestled on a pile of what could be hamster bedding. It nearly took my breath away, the lengths I had gone to in order to preserve the perfection of this imperfect thing. I relieved it of all wrappings and took it into the bathroom, where I let it fall from my hand and tumble to the tiled floor below. I'm not sure what I expected to happen, maybe a high pitched smash or wind-chime tinkling of shards, but it sounded more like an explosion. It boomed and resonated in the small echoing space, sending pieces flying in all directions of the floor. Not so perfect anymore.

I gathered up the pieces, scooping them into the wooden box carefully. I brought them back to my desk and began arranging them on the surface, like a sadistic 3D jigsaw. Over the next two hours, I glued the pot back together as best I could, at times sticking my fingers to its surface or to themselves or to the desk. I contemplated the true nature of imperfection as the pieces failed to stay together. I cut the tip of my middle finger and added blood to the glue. There was a hole in the side of the pot where a piece was missing, and I had no idea where it could have gone. The base of the pot had a sharp crease down it, which meant it no longer stood up without support. There were very few smooth surfaces anymore.

The Japanese call this the art of kintsugi, repairing broken ceramics with gold. I didn't have any gold glue, but like a good gay, I had a jar of glitter lying around, which was added to the mix. The pot sat there, propped against the box, broken and dazzling and cracked and incomplete and sparkling. I had bits of glitter stuck to my fingers and dusting my clothes. I started to see what imperfection actually felt like, and it was quite beautiful. I keep this now very Imperfect Pot on a shelf, in full view. It's a great conversation starter. Something that has surprised me, although maybe it's not that unusual, is that queer people seem to relate to it more deeply, or at least more quickly. There's something in us that resonates with the imperfect pot.

QUESTIONS TO PONDER

What experiences did you have growing up that have shaped your current outlook on life?

Which parts of your story still sting when you think about them?

What has helped you heal yourself so far?

What's your relationship to wholeness?

WHOLE

CONNECTING TO YOUR WHOLENESS

This activity will help you explore your connection to wholeness. It is based on the Japanese principles of wabi-sabi and kintsugi, which, as we've discussed, mainly use ceramics or pottery as the vehicle. For this, you can use anything. The task here is to shatter something. To fracture its wholeness. You might do this by:

- Ripping up a sheet of paper into many pieces
- Blowing up and bursting a balloon
- Smashing a mug
- Plucking the petals from a flower
- Throwing eggs against a wall

Obviously, make sure it's safe to break the thing you're about to experiment on. Don't smash anything that isn't yours, and don't do anything that might cause you damage – I'm all for the drama but I don't want anyone bleeding because of this book. You can take your time with this process over several days, or power through it all at once. The choice is yours.

Method

1. Choose the item you are about to shatter. Give yourself time to understand it – a minute, an hour or a week.

2. Contemplate its wholeness. That might mean revisiting it regularly, holding it close, or looking at it from across the room. Feel its textures and shape. Does it have a smell? If you hold it to your ear, what do you hear? What does it sound like indoors compared to outside? Take it in from different angles, in different types of light, at different times of day. What emotional quality does the item hold for you, if any? Does it have flexibility or rigidity? Can it be stretched or folded? How might it feel to know it is about to be shattered?
3. At the end of your period of contemplation, take your item to a shattering place. That might be exactly where you are standing, or somewhere outside or otherwise safer to do the deed.
4. Give the item a name. You might call it "wholeness" or "perfection", or something more specific, like "queerness" or "relationships" or "shame". Anything is fine, so long as it holds some meaning for you.
5. If you have the equipment, film yourself doing the shattering. Even better, film it in slow motion.
6. Just before, during and after the shattering takes place, what do you notice in yourself? What feelings come up? How is it to destroy the wholeness of something?
7. Once the shattering event has happened, collect all the pieces into one container.
8. Give yourself time to contemplate the object in its new state. Shake it. Listen to the sounds it makes. Does it feel different? What might its use be now?
9. When you're ready, take the item to a repairing place. That might be a desk or table, your bed or a kitchen surface. Using any materials you like, try to put the object back together again, so it resembles its original form as closely as possible.
10. To help your thinking, you could record yourself doing the rebuilding. Talk out loud about how this makes you feel. Why did you choose the materials you're using for the repair? What do you notice in the speed at which you work? Do any

feelings of joy or frustration or boredom come up? What is the point of repairing the item?

11. Once rebuilt, consider the new wholeness of the object. In what ways is the object still whole, even though it has been through that transformation? In which ways has something been lost? Are there ways in which it's even better than it was before?

What were the results of your experiment? Make a sketch or some notes here.

SHATTERED WHOLENESS IS STILL WHOLENESS

As queer people, we know exactly who we are. We also know that the possibility of being fully ourselves is our right. But over the course of our lives, people have tried to shatter the part of our wholeness that holds our queerness. Growing up in a heteronormative society can lead us to cover up the parts of ourselves that might bring trouble or cause us pain. So, our senses of wholeness may have picked up some cracks along with way, but those cracks don't make us break – they become part of the whole. Those looking at us will see what we want to show them, but when we come back to us, to our wholeness, it can feel fractured.

The lifelong adventure of finding, remembering, discovering and loving our wholeness takes deliberate attention, especially when we have to exist in a world of oppression that litters our path at every stage of our lives. Nevertheless, we all have a hidden whole at the deepest level of ourselves, and we know that our sexuality doesn't need to be fixed.

The world was not designed for queer people. We are not the default. Human brains seek out threats all the time. Most are calibrated like smoke detectors that sense when a proverbial fire is starting and blare to wake us up and save our lives. Some of us have oversensitive, queer smoke detectors that go off when the threat is miniscule, or when there is no threat at all. Walking along the street, my queer smoke detector starts wailing if I see a group of football lads coming toward me. I'll usually cross the road to keep it quiet.

I don't believe wholeness necessarily means completeness. For me, wholeness is not an end point because it's dynamic and always in a state of evolution. Wholeness is unshakeable, malleable and transforming. Wholeness gives us the opportunity to reimagine new futures. To reinvent ourselves and re-tell the stories that no longer serve us.

Imagine one of those football lads in the distance, on his phone, walking obliviously toward me, clipping my elbow, causing his phone to fall from his hand and tumble to the ground. He picks it up, face furious until he looks at my face. A soft smile breaks out on his. "Hi, sorry, I was miles away," he says. "Do I know you from somewhere? You look familiar. Maybe not. Anyway, I hope you have a good day." He smiles and walks away. A few minutes later, he sends me a message on Grindr: "Fancy a drink?"

Connecting to my wholeness gives me the chance to believe all kinds of possibilities instead of immediately jumping to worst-case scenarios. Wholeness is a limitless source of empowerment waiting to be remembered and used.

QUESTIONS TO PONDER

What are the stories you tell yourself about yourself that no longer serve you?

What is the story you'd love to live?

What ending do you want to write for yourself?

AGEING QUEERLY

“I came out much later, and in my language, there is nothing that describes lesbian or gay, bisexual, transgender. If you can't name something, you can't talk about it, and if you do talk about it, it may be in quite a derogatory way. You end up suppressing a part of who you don't even know yet.”

– PHYLL, 49

What's it like being your age? Ageing means different things to everyone.

. . . .

. . . .

. . . .

. . . .

. . . .

. . . .

. . . .

. . . .

. . . .

. . . .

. . . .

Ageing is inevitable, hopefully. It's one of those paradoxes where time plays tricks on the mind. As a child, I could not wait to be older, and now, the older I get, the faster time seems to go. I have spent ridiculous amounts of money on moisturizers, facials and Botox – not as a way of stopping time, but of looking less ... old – and yet, I love being able to age. It is a privilege not afforded to everyone, particularly queer people who came before us.

The process of ageing is both individual and collective. We all go through the physical changes that are influenced by our genes and the ongoing molecular disintegration happening in our bodies every day. More subjectively, our environment and how we live our lives also impact how we age. When seen through a medical lens, ageing is a gradual and inevitable process that results in a decline of physical and mental capabilities. Thanks, science.

There are things we can do to make ageing a little smoother, like eating well, and getting lots of sleep and having good social connections. If we can, we might move our bodies more. Despite the seemingly impossible number of hairs that now grow on the backs of my ears, and the creaky knees, back twinges and forgetful moments, ageing is an overwhelmingly positive experience for me. I have found and embraced a sense of freedom in my 50s that I'm greatly enjoying. It's not just the "I care less about what people think" cliché, although there's an element of that present, but more a bone-deep sense of solidity in my idea of self. It's not something that ossifies my ability to move or express myself; I can only compare it to a sturdy concrete platform from which I could launch a rocket.

If we follow the fantasy of what is considered "normal" ageing, where we avoid fatal diseases and go gracefully into the dying light, we may reach an ending that is not necessarily happy, but at least it might be pleasant. More likely, we will encounter one or more significant, life-changing illnesses that gradually affect our ability to move or think.

In middle age, we are not past the point of no return yet, but the horizon may feel closer than before. In the sweet absence of physical disease, we may encounter more social diseases, such as ageism and homophobia, that affect our overall wellness.

Older LGBTQ+ people often experience higher rates of mental illness in comparison to straight people of a similar age. Our community has a bigger incidence of anxiety, depression, substance use and suicidal thoughts. While those are not necessarily an inevitable result of ageing, they are within arm's reach for many queer folk because of how people treat us.

WHAT AGEING CAN MEAN FOR QUEER PEOPLE

Older LGBTQ+ people are more likely to live alone, without the support of children, which can mean more of a reliance on partners and friends who may themselves be experiencing similar changes from getting older. Many people in the LGBTQ+ community express worries about the possibility of having to live in a care home with predominantly heterosexual residents and staff.

Despite, and maybe because of, these factors, older LGBTQ+ folk are incredibly resilient. Many of us are living longer, healthier and happier with strong community connections. The time we are in now is the beginning of an explosion of older LGBTQ+ folk who will require access to health and care services that treat us exactly as we want to be treated. We are the first generation to be able to live truthfully and authentically ourselves, so the social and healthcare services really have to start thinking about how they will support this emerging generation of people who need their help in ways they have not experienced before.

HOW WE PERCEIVE MIDDLE AGE

As well as the physical and psychological shifts that happen as we get older, it can also be a time of existential and philosophical reflection. Aristotle said that middle age is the time when people can exercise their best virtue and reason (although he was a little lacking in his own advice when he got a bit judgy about gay people). Thomas Aquinas, another problematic homophobe, suggested that middle-aged folk could find joy in the pursuit of virtue. (To me, not being homophobic is a good example of having high morals, so again, maybe Tommy should taste a bit of his own medicine.)

During the Enlightenment of the 17th and 18th centuries, people like John Locke thought that middle age was a good time to give back to society (although his views on debauchery and a rejection of sodomy may lead us to believe he didn't mean giving back in that way). Immanuel Kant also believed that midlife was a time to further personal and collective enlightenment through ethical behaviour (but sadly – do you see any patterns here? – he excluded homosexuals from that category as he thought we were immoral and disrespectful). What a Kant.

Isn't it fascinating that so many of the people who said the most about ageing also used their platforms to take a pop at folk like us? Thankfully, they are now dead, and we are still here (still queer), with new generations of queer philosophers and thinkers who can contribute so much more to the discussion on ageing.

Judith Butler talks about how performative gender identity is a factor of how we perceive and experience our middle age, as we are often in conflict with societal expectations of what it means to be a person. Butler argues that one's identity, which includes age, is never fixed, but always in a state of change, over which we have some control.

Thinkers like Kathryn Bond Stockton and Jack Halberstam take the idea of queer ageing even further with concepts like "queer time", which rejects the linear heteronormative timeline of ageing. Instead, queer time allows us the choice of ageing in whatever ways we wish, fitting our uniquely queer experiences. They label straight ageing expectations as "chrono-normativity", which sounds not only very cool, but also like something Janeway and the crew of Voyager would rightfully avoid on their journey through the Delta quadrant. Halberstam suggests that getting older as a queer person can be a time of further liberation, not decline, characterized by ongoing exploration and experimentation with our own personal narratives. I'm here for that.

It is exciting to me that a whole new theory of queer ageing is emerging. It comes not a moment too soon. We no longer have to sit back while homophobes write about us. We can shape our own futures, develop new ways of looking at life and create exciting realities for ourselves. One way to do this is through sharing our stories, which helps us make sense of the world.

QUESTIONS TO PONDER

How has your sense of self changed with age?

What is on your mind more as you get older?

What would people who knew you a long time ago say if they met you now?

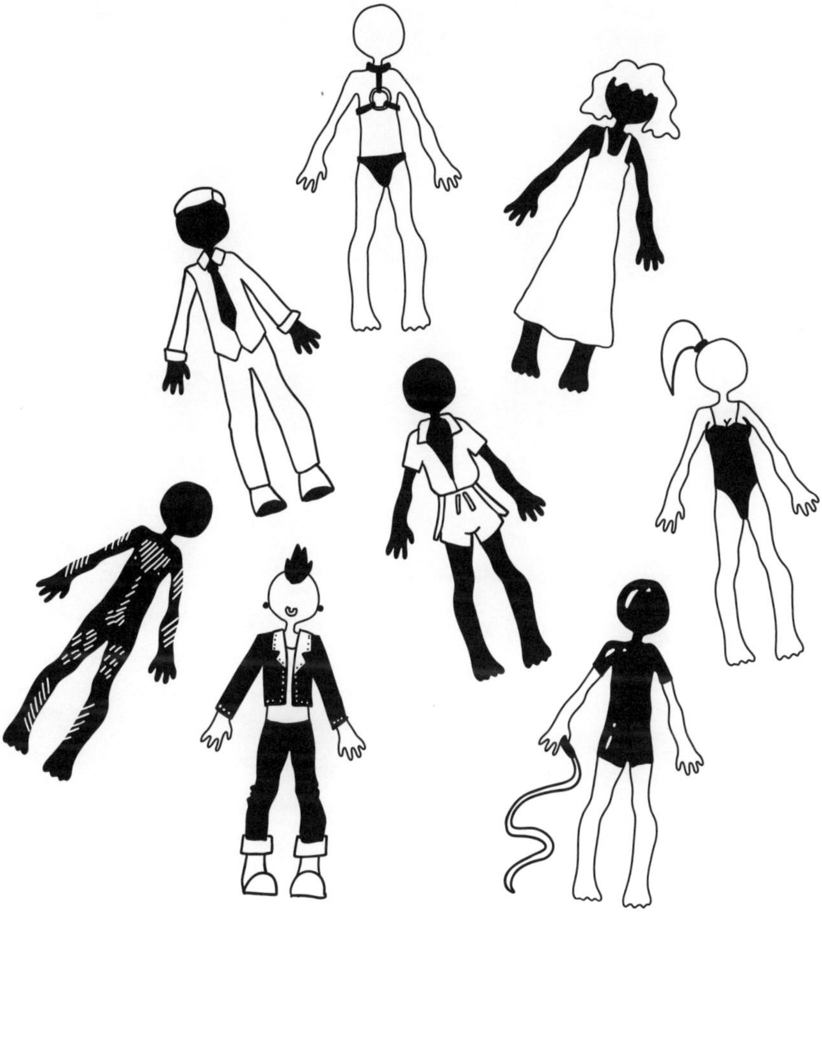

SHARING STORIES

> “Whenever people tell me I can’t do something, well, I do it anyway. I’m etching and creating a life for myself regardless of what other people think.”
>
> – LIZ, 58

We all have our own unique narrative to our lives, but how understood do you usually feel?

Aren't stories brilliant? Throughout this book are quotes from the people I interviewed while researching this work. Queer voices are vital. I was struck by the overwhelming amount of straight people who have made their way into print discussing the human condition and how we might better ourselves. The queer voices in this space are present but totally outnumbered, drowned out in a cacophony of heteronormativity. We will never, nor should we, silence those straight voices. We just need to listen more carefully and closely to those of us who may be lost in the noise. Our experiences are powerful, different and valid. They deserve to be heard.

So many people gave me their time and stories with generosity and vulnerability. As a community, our tapestry is rich and colourful. The folk who shared their experiences with me can be summed up as deeply reflective, resilient and diverse. They – we – have lived through significant social, cultural and personal shifts. Our stories reflect the complexities of our lives in all their beautiful and difficult hues. The people who opened their worlds to me are to be celebrated and commended. The willingness of people to contribute their stories, experiences and wisdom to this work is truly humbling. And, as I explained earlier, they inspired me to include some of my own stories from childhood to the present day as a way of illustrating the themes and ideas that emerged from the wider conversations.

Much has been said about the power of vulnerability. Despite knowing this intellectually, I find it hard to be vulnerable and show my soft, fuzzy places. As you will see in the pages to come, I believe myself to be resilient and competent, traits that emerged during a childhood often characterized by chaos and difficulty. My response to that was not to fold in on myself, but to strengthen my ability to survive and exist, to make something of my life and find peace and happiness. This has pros and cons. The cost of this way of being is often a refusal to ask for help or admit when I am not feeling okay. I find it hard to ask for what I want or need, and even when someone else asks what they can do for me, I find it equally impossible to articulate. I would not change anything about my life experiences, as they have made me who I am now, but there have been hard lessons to live with, and I am sure more will come my way. I hope they do. I'm not done changing yet.

QUESTIONS TO PONDER

Who really knows your story?

What aspects of your life do you keep to yourself?

Who makes you feel most able to be the most honest version of you?

WHAT'S YOUR STORY?

"I went out clubbing with some friends, and this is the last time I took any sort of drugs. I was quite high. We went into this bar with a drag queen on the stage, and as we went in, she was calling for volunteers, and I just ran up and got on the stage. She announced this dance-off, and I was dancing, and I jumped into the splits and burst a testicle. I didn't even know this was a possibility, but because I was so high, I didn't know it happened."

– PHIL, 42

Think back to the beginning of your queer story: when did you first meet another queer person?

. . . .

. . . .

. . . .

. . . .

. . . .

. . . .

. . . .

. . . .

. . . .

. . . .

This is the first self-help book aimed at midlife LGBTQ+ people that recognizes we are whole, powerful and capable of joy, without the need for acceptance or to change who we are. I am surprised it has taken this long for a book like this to arrive, but I'm also not at all shocked. There are millions of middle-aged queer people in the world. That's a lot of sore backs. Our relationship as a human race to our sexuality is, as they might say, complicated. You would think that after existing for a few million years we would be more evolved when it comes to our sexualities, but here we are in the 21st century, still freaking out about boys kissing boys, girls kissing girls and some kissing both.

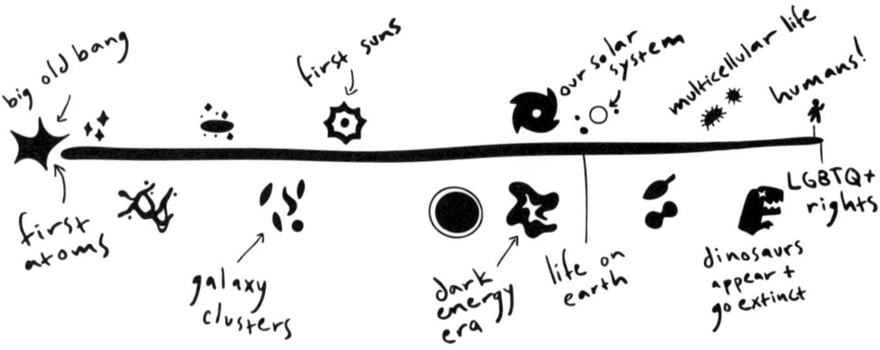

I like to imagine neanderthal lesbians watching the sun set over Dinosaur Mountain, huddled by the fire, bellies full of leaf tea, nuts and berries. I picture queer throuples in the Scottish Highlands in the time of Robert the Bruce, drinking peaty whisky together on cold winter nights. Or I conjure images of husbands in the 1600s choosing frock coats for the summer festival. Although imagined, each scenario is plausible because we have always been here. It's just that nobody wanted to talk about us, or if they did, it was in negative ways. More often than not, queer people don't have children, so maybe we just ran out of people to tell our stories through time, but we have still somehow always managed to be woven through the fabric of our societies and cultures.

Those of us born in the 1970s and '80s lived through a unique snapshot of time. In our case, so many stories of those like us who came before us were unfortunately lost, twisted or invented to suit the politics, religion and fashion of the day. I grew up hearing very little about queer people, and those who were mentioned rarely had happy endings. I have been led to believe that in the long line of my family tree, I was the first and only gay person. In the whole history of time, they say it's just me. But that simply cannot be true. While I like the "queen supreme" status within my family, it's both narcissistic and impossible to believe that I was the first. My family can be traced back to the dawn of time if you try hard enough. I am not the only one. Of course, life has changed a lot since the neanderthal days. Printing presses, then cameras and now TikTok have made it so much easier to see representations of ourselves than braving a woolly mammoth-inhabited tundra to check out a cave painting by the local queer artist.

In the 21st century, we have access to every flavour of sexuality we choose, with new ones being revealed all the time. When I was ten, it was a huge treat to get an ice cream from Casa Marcini, an Italian gelateria in my hometown of Aberdeen. My favourite flavour was pear – so exotic and different from the traditional block of yellow vanilla I was used to. In those days, there were gays and lesbians, none of this fancy bisexuality stuff, and certainly nobody I knew had ever met anyone who proudly defined themselves as queer. In fact, being called queer was the worst thing that could be said about you. Now, in the 2020s, I can enjoy a vegan matcha gelato on Old Compton Street while chatting with my pansexual transmasculine friend. Ten-year-old me would have understood the words "street" and "friend" in that sentence. The point is, things change. We evolve and expand.

I like imagining new futures. Nostalgia, to me, is a prison. I don't enjoy looking behind and certainly don't wish we could go back to any kind of good old days. In politics, around the time of a general election in the UK, it fills me with dread when I hear that a party "will bring back" anything. It usually comes from a lack of imagination and a fetishization of something that probably didn't work before, but people like it because of the comfort and familiarity of the well-worn path. I much prefer the road less travelled. Or do I? Maybe it's just the only road that was ever available to me. I was – as well as, apparently, the only gay person in the history of my family – the first of my family to get any kind of qualifications at school. I was the first to leave Aberdeen and go to university. I was the first to get a master's degree and the only one to get a doctorate.

They are markers of a very specific kind of achievement, and I don't believe they make me any better or worse than anyone else, but the further into education I went, the farther I felt from my family. Encouraging words are great, but they can also feel empty when the person offering them has no actual understanding of the situation because they have never had to go through it themselves. When I told my dad, two-thirds through my doctorate, that I was really struggling, he said, "You'll be fine, you always are," which is both true to him and massively false to me. Being the first of anything is a blessing and a curse. As the first gay person to exist in my family, not only had nobody else ever experienced what it was like to be queer, the message was very different. In that context, I was told I definitely would not be fine.

A SNAPSHOT OF MY STORY

Growing up in the 1970s and '80s meant the following things for me:

- At 17, I first met another openly gay person. No straight person can ever say they hadn't met someone like them before their late teens.
- The sensationalized coverage of AIDS in the media led me to believe I would be dead by 30, and not only would it be my own fault, it would be God's punishment for my deviant lifestyle.

- Kids at my school used my sexuality as a reason to bully me, and I couldn't tell anyone how they were treating me. A double whammy of silence.
- I kept a secret diary where I wrote about the men I fancied.
- Teachers at my school were not allowed to talk about homosexuality in any positive sense, if at all, because of Section 28 of the Local Government Act.
- Any attempt at having sex with another man in my late teens would have been illegal due to the age of consent for gay men being 21.
- Characters on TV who were coded gay were objects of ridicule, pity, celibacy and freakery.
- Our Prime Minister at the time, Margaret Thatcher, said with horror that children were growing up believing they had an inalienable right to be gay.
- The *Daily Mail* reported on an exciting development for potential parents when the "gay gene" was almost discovered, as it meant queer foetuses could in the future be aborted.
- I was warned that I should never get into a car with a strange man because older homosexuals were predators who like to recruit and convert young boys.
- People called me a bummer before I knew what bumming was.
- Being gay saved my life.

This section of the book – Part I: "Still Here!" – is about locating ourselves in the present by understanding our past. It took thousands of words to get to the statement that "being gay saved my life". I have no doubt that my queerness was an accelerant, a propellant, that got me out of Aberdeen. My difference acted as a catalyst for change that took me away from home to create a new home and live by my own rules.

I am so grateful to be gay. I thank whichever deities blessed me with my sexuality because it gives me such joy. I've never been someone who says they don't want their sexuality to define them. Mine totally does, along with so many other elements that make me who I am. Allowing my sexuality to define me has given me empathy, humility and an utter refusal to let anyone stand in my way who believes me to be less than a straight person. I did not choose to be gay. I am just fortunate that I am.

QUESTIONS TO PONDER

What happened when you first came out to yourself?

Who were your champions when you came out? Who held you back?

Think about the era in which you were a child or teenager. What did growing up during this time mean for you?

WRITING YOUR OWN STORY

"I used to think I didn't have a story worth telling. But I think I do."

– JEREMY, 45

What patterns of behaviour have you carried for too long?

Claim your own narrative

As queer people, so many of the stories people tell about us are untrue, hurtful or both. If we are able to hold those stories up to the light and inspect their utility in middle age, we can check if they are useful or not. Choosing to exclude other people's opinions from our own thoughts and beliefs can be so useful in claiming our own narratives. It helps us to locate ourselves. At times, I can do this deliberately and thoughtfully. Sometimes it comes as a complete surprise.

I felt my age recently while I was having a chat with a friend, talking about our coming-out experiences. He said, "I don't know about you, but my biggest fear as a teenager was always that someone would see my dating profile online, screenshot it and send it to my parents." I smiled when I said, "When I was a teenager, the internet wasn't invented." Condensing our lives into a story can feel challenging. After all, we have a lot of material by this stage. You might consider the timeline of events that you've lived through that has brought you here. For me, it starts with *Clash of the Titans.*

Born a crime

In 1861 in the UK, the death penalty for homosexual acts was repealed, replaced by a prison sentence between ten years and life. That law stayed in place for the next 94 years. In 1967, homosexuality (in private, between two men over the age of 21) was decriminalized in England. Six years later in 1973, in Aberdeen, Scotland, I was born. The first seven years of my life were lived illegally because Scotland only decriminalized homosexuality in 1980. I was always gay. I was born a crime. In 1981, finally legal, at the age of eight, I watched *Clash of the Titans*. If you haven't seen this film – it's a classic – it's the story of Perseus battling the demons of Greek mythology. The film stars Harry Hamlin, who spends most of his time topless or in a toga, and on seeing him, I immediately knew I was gay, at the deepest level of my soul from brain to body. That year also marked the first recorded case of AIDS in the UK, just as I had come out to myself.

I was outed by my parents at 15, when they read my diary and discovered I was in love with George Michael. (If you need a reason, watch the "Club Tropicana" video, all I'll say is Speedos.) George Michael was outed ten years after I was, but at the time of my "coming out", I didn't know a single other gay person in the world. That happened in 1988, the same year Margaret Thatcher's government introduced Section 28, making it illegal for teachers to talk positively, or at all, about homosexuality in schools. Instead, we were shown educational videos about the dangers of AIDS, while my friends in the class laughed and called it the gay plague, throwing around slurs like "bummer" and "poofter" for good measure. I had not so much as kissed anyone at that point, but I assumed this was now my fate. This was what happened to gay people, and I would be dead by the time I was 30.

In 1991, I moved to London. At that time, the World Health Organization still classed homosexuality as a mental disorder. Freddie Mercury announced he had AIDS and died the next day. I was 17, and it was illegal for me to have sex, as the age of consent for gay men was 21. In 1994, the year of my 21st birthday, the government voted against equalizing the age of consent, instead reducing it to 18 for gay men. So, at least I wasn't a criminal anymore.

In 2000 I met Dan, the love of my life. That year, Section 28 was repealed in Scotland, but not in England. It was also the year that, in England, the age of consent was finally equalized to 16 for everyone. LGBTQ+ people were still not allowed to join the armed forces, though. It was still legal in the UK for someone to lose their job because they were gay. In 2005, my best friend of 20 years announced she was getting married to her boyfriend in Fiji. When looking at travel details, it became clear that if my partner and I went to the wedding and shared a room, there was a chance we might be arrested. So, we missed the wedding. (Fijian law has since changed, but in 2002, they created a new law to explicitly make same-sex marriage illegal.) In 2010, after being together for a decade, Dan and I had a civil partnership ceremony in Scotland. It was illegal for us to get married at that point. In 2017, on Dan's 40th birthday, we went back to Scotland to convert our civil partnership to a marriage, although it was still illegal for us to marry in a church.

In 2017, Dan and I joined a new gym. I was excited because the membership card was the first official document with my new married name on it. When leaving the gym one day, the guy on reception called me over and said, "Someone found your brother's membership card in a locker." I told him he must be mistaken, as I don't have a brother. He apologized, saying he made an assumption because we had the same surname. I told him Dan was my husband. I often wonder why he guessed brother before husband.

Last year, I changed my mobile phone contract. On the call, the salesperson asked if I needed another line, maybe a new phone for my wife. I told him that my husband didn't need a new phone, thank you very much. This year Dan and I will have been together 26 years. If we were to celebrate abroad, there are still 68 countries in the world we couldn't visit in case we are imprisoned.

In the years since 2020, it has felt increasingly like open season on the queer community. In January 2023, over 200,000 people signed a petition for schools in the UK to remove LGBTQ+ content from relationship education. The government's response was that they didn't have to include it anyway. At the start of February 2024, after voting to recognize same-sex blessings in church, the Archbishop of Canterbury said, "For the first time, the Church of England will publicly, unreservedly and joyfully welcome same-sex couples in church," but the General Synod voted against performing weddings in church. The Archbishop also said he would "rather see the church lose its privileged status as the established church of the country than risk fracturing it over same-sex marriage". The US Government kicked off 2025 by rolling back legislation that protected LGBTQ+ people from discrimination, banning pride flags from public buildings and waging war on Diversity, Equity and Inclusion in organizations. It is a scary time, and the United Kingdom is following quickly behind our American cousins. It feels increasingly dangerous to be out and proud.

In my fifth decade – my golden jubilee – in so many ways, despite so many things, I feel golden. I am happy, I have my health, I feel proud of who I am. I feel lucky to be here, to be shining. I hope it lasts. I often think about getting older. What if something happens to me and I have to go into a straight nursing home? Sometimes I think about how Dan or I will cope when one of us dies. There isn't yet a legally recognized word for a man whose husband has died (heteronormative couples get "widow" or "widower"). I wonder how we will be able to talk about and process that moment when, right now, there is no language for it.

It has been more than four decades since I watched *Clash of the Titans*, and I feel like I've been battling my own mythological demons since. In my whole story, there are very few moments when I have ever directly experienced homophobia. Instead, it is like debris in the water I swim in, something to navigate and notice. I've lived through periods of depression and anxiety, and I've come to see mental well-being as something fragile and soft that needs to be looked after. But I'm here, and I'm thriving.

Compassion begins with kindness to ourselves. Forgiveness. Love. For despite all the people, directly or indirectly, who have told me I am wrong for being who I am, I have never once thought there was anything wrong with me. Despite living in an atmosphere of prejudice, I have always known I am okay, and it's them who have the problem.

The world is often not very compassionate to us as queer people. It makes it even more important that we are compassionate to ourselves, and to each other. When we start really seeing and believing our own worth, recognizing that we are whole, we cultivate a stronger sense of self-esteem and confidence. We feel empowered as we confidently navigate and overcome everyday barriers and challenges. This helps us foster hope and growth within, and finally find the strength to effectively help and lead others.

So, what's your story? Imagine your life is to be turned into a film.

- What is the title?

- Which famous actor would play you?
- Is it an indie word-of-mouth flick or a huge blockbuster?
- What genre is the movie?
- What is the message under the narrative?
- Where has there been a plot twist?
- Who appears in the credits?
- Who would sing the theme song?
- Are you the hero or the villain?
- What is the strap line on the poster?

Draw the poster here:

There's power in claiming our own narratives. The story so far is not the ending. Knowing how we came to this place can help us write the next scene of our lives. Knowing where we have come from gives us clues and signs of what shaped us to become who we are. We can't change the past, but we can learn from it and take action in the present that will shape the future. Every day is an opportunity to change the script.

QUESTIONS TO PONDER

What are the landmark moments in your life that have helped you be more you?

Who might you need to forgive for not knowing better?

Where do you hold anger, sadness or regret?

WHERE ARE WE NOW?

> " I'm on PrEP now, in an open relationship. The generation before us could not have sex without consequences. The younger generation can have sex without the ultimate consequence. That is different from our age. I do wonder whether our age group is almost having a second wind."
>
> – IAN, 48

Getting to know where we are in our life is pivotal to finding our wholeness. Knowing where we came from, who we are and how we got to this place begins the process of learning new information about ourselves.

Arriving in midlife is the end of the first part of our life journey. We each have our own unique lifelines stretching behind us, shaped by a world that is changing all the time. Maybe some of our wholeness has been chipped or cracked along the way, but we have made it to this midpoint. It's a time to pause, reflect and take stock.

The next part of our work together is to examine different aspects of what it means to be a middle-aged queer person, highlighting any particular areas to which you might want to pay special attention and maybe even make some changes.

So where are you in your life journey now? What is "now" like?

QUESTIONS TO PONDER

What are some things about you in the present that are to be celebrated?

. . . .

. . . .

. . . .

. . . .

. . . .

. . . .

What did you think life would be like at this stage?

. . . .

. . . .

. . . .

. . . .

. . . .

. . . .

What is going on in your life at the moment that helps or hinders your wholeness?

. . . .

. . . .

. . . .

. . . .

. . . .

. . . .

. . . .

THE QUEER WHEEL OF MIDLIFE

> "That's always a fear: am I going to be in an old-age home and nobody's going to come and I'm going to be super depressed and be like, 'Oh my god, I have nothing, no purpose'?"
>
> – MIKE S, 48

What did you want to be when you grew up and how has that worked out?

. . . .

. . . .

. . . .

. . . .

. . . .

. . . .

. . . .

. . . .

. . . .

. . . .

. . . .

REINVENTING OURSELVES

When I was a kid, I wanted to be an astronaut, a pharmacist or a member of a boy band. Quite different career choices. Given I have terrible eyesight, an awful memory and, according to my husband, "the singing voice of Kermit in a blender", none of those career paths were particularly attainable. In my actual career history, I've been a mushroom picker, shop assistant, prison psychologist, care assistant, head of HR and a coach. That list is not exhaustive. I refuse to believe I just have to be one thing for the rest of my life, in work and all other aspects too. I was born Mr Paul Taylor, and I will die Dr Paul Taylor-Pitt. I have been fat, thin, a smoker, a drinker, a non-smoker, a non-drinker, a marathon runner, a podcaster, long-haired, no-haired, blank-skinned and tattooed. All the while, I have always been me. None of my reinventions have ever changed who I am, unless I had the gift of being changed by them. I hope I never stop changing, or growing, for as long as possible. I am sure there will come a time in my (hopefully) old age when I decide, that's it, fuck this, I will be this way for the rest of my days, but I am far away from that point today. Madonna recently did some promotion where she used the line, "I keep reinventing myself so I can keep being myself," and my mind exploded. It made so much sense. The only way I can keep being me is to constantly change what it means to be this person.

The boundaries of my personality might be pretty fixed, but the rest is up for grabs. It goes against the idea that we are one thing and to go beyond that is difficult, particularly if we are over 30. You can't teach an old dog new tricks, but people can learn new tricks until the day we die. I don't believe in regrets either (even when the questionable things I've done haunt me just as I am falling asleep). In other words, everything I have ever done has led me to this point. If anything, any single choice, had been different, I would not be here right now.

What if where I am isn't where I want to be, though? Could I find the grace to be kind to that truth? To know that this is a step on a bigger stairway, and my eventual destination would not be possible without being right here, right now. Every moment we are alive, we are changing. We can't stop it even if we wanted to. What if we put all of that relentless change to good use?

LOOKING FORWARD

When I reach points of stuck-ness, I take myself somewhere quiet and stay very still. I try to hear sounds close by and far away. I feel the weight of my body on the ground. I listen for my heartbeat. It reminds me that even when I am not moving, my body is in motion. If I hold my breath my heart still beats. It helps to release something that might be blocking what I want to do. I do have a certain tendency to be stubborn and want to get my own way, neither of which are always particularly sexy qualities, but the upside of them is that I can be incredibly determined, focused and deliberate in where I put my energy. Don't get me wrong, I can get lost in an Instagram Reels hole for hours if I let myself, but it's by choice. If I don't allow my brain to cool down now and again, I sometimes think it might spark itself on fire. I run very hot. I wasn't always like this, and perhaps it is another unexpected outcome of this midlife era. I feel like there is no time to waste anymore.

My mum died when she was 53, one year older than I am now. One grandfather died at 56 and the other at 60. These numbers are not big. When I think of how fast the past ten years has gone by, if the next ten go just as quick, I'll be celebrating another big birthday before the glow wears off the last one. So, I have to ask myself ...

- Who do I want to be over this next decade as I age out of midlife?
- How do I want to be, to act, to live?
- In what ways do I want people to experience me when we have time together?

I'm sure in the past I've been described as moody and unpredictable, boring and selfish. I hope I've also been seen as kind, generous, funny and lovable. Instead of painting myself into a corner of who I want to be, I would like to believe I will always be someone who is curious about the world and how it works. Maybe understanding that better I might effect some positive change.

Who will you be today? This afternoon? In an hour? Right now? If you were to reinvent yourself for 20 minutes and try a new way of being that you've always fancied experiencing, who might you experiment with? You don't have to stick with it forever – you don't have to stick with anything. You have infinite possibilities inside you that require no money, resources or equipment to play with. All you need is energy, a bit of time and the courage to say, "Fuck it, let's give this a go."

QUESTIONS TO PONDER

What does the idea of reinventing yourself bring up for you?

....

....

....

....

Who would you be if you no longer believed negative stories about yourself?

....

....

....

....

What might it look like if you were able to be ten per cent more you? Twenty per cent?

....

....

....

....

....

What does the best version of you look and feel like?

....

....

....

....

....

INTRODUCING THE QUEER WHEEL OF MIDLIFE

> “I feel resigned to being single. I am resigned to feeling a little bit alienated from my community. I don’t know when it happened, but inadvertently people my age have been edged out of the gay scene.”
>
> – JOHNNY, 60

How is middle age working out for you so far?

. . . .

. . . .

. . . .

. . . .

. . . .

. . . .

. . . .

. . . .

. . . .

. . . .

This section introduces The Queer Wheel of Midlife, a tool for self-coaching based on themes from the conversations I had with the middle-aged queer folk who generously shared their stories.

When I'm working with a coaching client, they often don't know what they want to work on at first. The topic emerges in time, and we go with whatever feels important in the moment. Offering space, silence and sometimes a question or two can help the process move forward. Obviously, I'm not there with you as you read this book, but I hope that it might feel like I am. This book is less self-help and more of what I like to call biblio-coaching.

BIBLIO-COACHING

Self-help implies a set of instructions and an expectation that you are on your own. But self-coaching is not quite right to describe this process, either. Coaching is a relationship where two people, coach and client, have a conversation together. Self-coaching implies you are both coach and client, which I am not sure is entirely possible unless you try some weird and wonderful role-playing – and, if that is your thing, more power to you. Instead, we could try a different way of describing the relationship between the words on the page and the hands holding them. Structured, supported biblio-coaching. I am attached to using the word "coaching", as it comes with principles and practices in a way that "help" doesn't. After all, coaching is a process through which you can follow your own agenda, exploring possibilities and making commitments to take action based on your new insights.

As with any model, I encourage you to use The Queer Wheel of Midlife where it works and ignore it where it doesn't. Change it, break it, upgrade it, make it your own.

If the themes speak to you, that's great. If any of them need to change to make it even more resonant, go ahead and adapt it. Those older and younger than us may have their own Queer Wheels of Life that emerge from their lived experiences and contexts. This one is by us midlife queers, for us, and can continue to evolve with us.

FROM US, FOR US

There are many good and helpful coaching models to explore, but most, if not all of them, come from a heteronormative perspective. Of course, that's not necessarily a bad thing. Many coaches from the LGBTQ+ community use those models with great success with their LGBTQ+ clients. If it works, it works. However, building a coaching model from the ground up gives us an opportunity to queer the coaching process based on our own experiences and expectations.

Take the Wheel of Life as an example. It has earned its place as one of the best known and commonly used coaching tools over the last six decades. It was created by Paul J. Meyer of the Success Motivation Institute, a (straight) giant in the personal development field. The Wheel of Life was designed as a visual aid to help people achieve a balance across a range of areas of their life, showing where they may have strengths and gaps. At the heart of it is purpose and meaning. The original Wheel of Life from 1960 covers eight areas:

1. Career and work
2. Finance
3. Health and wellness
4. Home and environment
5. Recreation and fun
6. Spirituality
7. Relationships
8. Personal development

Each of those areas are undoubtedly important and could be seen as universal. However, with so many middle-aged queer people sharing their stories with me for this book, I was able to bear witness to people's hopes, fears, dreams and preoccupations. The themes that emerged from those conversations lent themselves to a new model that felt congruent with who we are. While some of them overlapped with the traditional Wheel of Life topics, there was a significant difference in tone and breadth.

The following are the ten most common threads that connected all those conversations.

1. We hold incredible stories of LGBTQ+ identity and experiences

Our tales of growing up gay, coming out (or not), of self-discovery, relationships, sexuality, gender identity, internalized homophobia, stigma, discrimination, trauma, love, joy and hope have rarely been shared so openly. Our generation has unique experiences that are at risk of being lost if they are not captured, spoken or discussed.

2. Each of us has our own relationship to ageing, middle age and mortality

While reflections on turning 40, 50 or 60 differ, there are consistent themes on what it is like to age as a queer person. There are generational differences in our community that can make us feel isolated. We're also contemplating legacy, retirement planning, care homes and what it means to be emerging elders in the community.

3. We are navigating increasingly complex relationship dynamics

We start experiencing significant shifts in our relationships with parents, siblings and partners, seeing each other age and change – or not – and often becoming more marginalized in community. We may or may not have children who are also ageing, and we may also still be finding and redefining chosen families. Our marriages, singledom, desires, love and sex are often private or even secretive. We may have lived through divorce and bereavement, as well as domestic abuse and assault, often committed by those closest to us.

4. We live with fluctuating mental health and challenges to personal growth

Many of us have scars from growing up gay in a homophobic world. We may have experienced anxiety, self-doubt and imposter syndrome in different aspects of life. Some of us still suffer from people-pleasing, burnout and a lack of boundaries. Our self-confidence could be better. Therapy and counselling have helped in some cases. Others are still struggling.

5. Midlife is a place of big career and life transitions

We threw ourselves into our jobs as we were growing up, determined to make something of ourselves. We have made significant career changes, but maybe some of us have reached a point where we're seeking more meaning from work, while also feeling stuck and wrestling with the idea of finding purpose as we get closer to the end of our working lives.

6. Contemporary LGBTQ+ community and culture can be confusing

We may find ourselves on the margins of the community that we wish to belong to, feeling pressure to conform to standards or cultural norms. Many of us have moved away from the nightlife scene and find it hard to see a clear replacement. Generational gaps can make it difficult for us to be seen or feel like we belong.

7. We have lived through seismic changes in political, societal and cultural attitudes

We are a generation that grew up in analogue times before the internet, finding our way through an increasingly digital world in our middle age. We were brought up in a climate where homophobia and discrimination were everyday occurrences. We were perhaps not the first to be touched directly by HIV/AIDS, although many of us were, but we were entering our early adulthood in the shadow of prejudice and fear. In the UK, we saw the introduction of Section 28 and suffered through decades of right-wing government rule.

8. We don't talk enough about sex, sexuality and the type of relationships we want

Growing up with heteronormative expectations placed on us meant some of us found it hard to come out and be our authentic sexual selves. We were rarely, if ever, taught that sex can be pleasurable for queer people. Middle age is giving us opportunities for sexual self-discovery, exploring different relationship models: non-monogamy, open relationships, polyamory or marriage. Some of us feel stuck in our relationship patterns. Others struggle to find someone, particularly in the era of dating apps. Aspects of queer life, such as cruising, polyamory, fetish and kink, often remain hidden even from our closest friends.

9. Getting older means finding deeper truth in self-expression

For some of us, ageing has been an opportunity to leave behind the self-consciousness of our younger selves, exploring new and authentic ways of expressing our individuality. This includes fluidity around gender identity, talking about ourselves in a different and evolving language, and expressing our internal selves through our external appearance like tattoos, clothes and hair. We may be more confident and comfortable sharing our inner selves more visibly on the outside.

10. The pursuit of self-acceptance and authentic living is paramount

In midlife, many of us are taking deliberate and positive steps to release or come to terms with aspects of ourselves that held us back in the past. We are trying to let go of shame and stop people-pleasing; and in discovering who we want to become, we are taking decisive steps to find and belong to supportive communities where we can be supported in our quest to be true to ourselves.

Upon uncovering these themes, I knew it was time to reinvent the Wheel of Life, to "queer it up" and make it relevant to those of us in middle age. The Queer Wheel of Midlife is centred on wholeness. Each of the main areas contain further themes that can be explored. The Queer Wheel of Midlife is holistic, current and specific. It is, of course, incomplete, as all coaching models are, but hopefully everyone can relate to at least one of the factors that lend to wholeness. It is the beginning of a new conversation where we might hold the discussions we've always had up to the light and re-imagine them through a queer lens.

The Queer Wheel of Midlife explores our wholeness in relation to:

1. **Identity**: intersectionality, sexuality, race, gender, neurodiversity, religion, nationality
2. **Intimacy**: sex, friendships, boundaries, pleasure, relationship models, equality
3. **Mental wellbeing**: burnout, depression, anxiety, trauma, self-care, resilience
4. **Self-acceptance**: self-love, discovery, acceptance, shame, homonegativity, discrimination
5. **Self-expression**: image, authenticity, confidence, visibility, voice
6. **Belonging**: elderhood, parenting, representation, home, safe spaces, family
7. **Life transitions**: physical changes, marriage, divorce, retirement, career, finances, location
8. **Legacy**: being remembered or forgotten, impact, purpose
9. **Mortality**: loss, meaning, change, death

THE QUEER WHEEL OF MIDLIFE

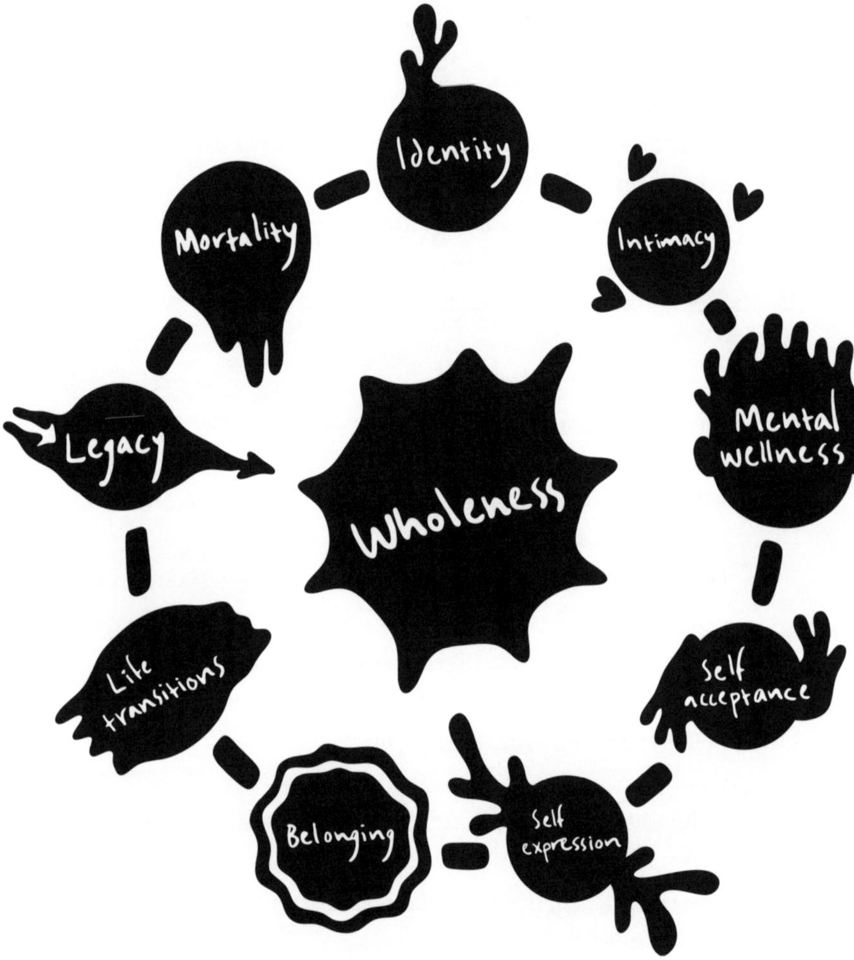

HOW TO USE THE QUEER WHEEL OF MIDLIFE

> "I can't tell you if I was bullied because I was autistic, because I was queer, because I was gender diverse, or because they're all the same thing. I don't actually think they are different things. I don't think they're discrete categories of meanness."
>
> – ASLAN, 48

Each of the nine themes is an enabler of, or barrier to, our wholeness. You are invited to consider each theme with the question "How near to or far from wholeness am I?" For each theme, give yourself a score on a scale from 1 to 5, where 1 is "very close to wholeness" and 5 is "very far from wholeness". For example, when I consider my identity, I have access to a lot of privilege as a white, cisgendered, able-bodied, western man with no religious affiliation. The only aspect of my identity that has caused an issue with my wholeness is my sexuality, and that is because of society's response to it rather than my own relationship to it. I would score my identity 3. On the other hand, when I consider intimacy, I remember that I still have some hang-ups where sex is concerned. The hangover of growing up in the homophobic 1970s and '80s, living through AIDS and the general stigma of "promiscuity" has left a scar on my sense of intimacy. I score it 4. Maybe even 5.

You can make a note on your scores at the end of each section. There's a blank wheel for you to fill at the end of the chapter.

Visually, my completed wheel looks quite jagged, more so than I expected. I can see where I feel like I'm doing quite well, particularly in relation to self-expression, belonging and identity. Areas I might need to keep a watchful eye on are mental wellness and belonging. Places where I would prioritize some deeper self-inquiry are intimacy, life transitions and mortality.

I don't believe the goal should ever be to reach perfection. It's not possible or even desirable. The Queer Wheel of Midlife should be a dynamic document that shifts with time, reflecting the changes that naturally occur as we age and grow. It is useful as a tool for noticing and prioritizing. It can help us work out where to start, and also where we might celebrate the progress we have already made.

To illustrate each section of The Queer Wheel of Midlife, I'm going to share some stories of my own experiences in each of the different areas. They are offered as embarrassing examples, funny tales and hopeful anecdotes that might inspire you to do some reflecting, writing or thinking as you work through your own version of The Queer Wheel of Midlife. All the stories are – for better or worse – true.

1. IDENTITY

The characteristics determining who or what a person or thing is

> "You start to etch away at your identity. And not even being conscious of it, because it's easier to be a duck when you're with ducks, as opposed to being a goose, right? Like, you're close enough but not the same. And you don't even realize you have started putting on duck feathers and trying to shrink yourself to be the size of a duck."
>
> – CHRISTIANNE, 45

I always swim in the slow lane of the pool. I know who I am. Even when it's peak time at the gym, I'm often the only person in the slow lane. Sometimes I'll be joined by a nice, smiley woman, but rarely another man. Men, particularly the straight ones, seem to have a huge problem with admitting they might be a slow swimmer. I'm not there to beat anything except my own desire to stay longer in bed, so it makes no difference to me which lane I'm in. Others seem determined to be fast even when they clearly aren't. I call it "toxic mascu-lane-ity" and feel smug at my own joke as I swim uninterrupted in what I now prefer to think of as "the honest lane".

I've always been allergic to inauthentic people. They make my skin itch. Fake people are not welcome in my life. I know everyone editorializes a little about aspects of their achievements – yes, I have eight O-Levels, but most of them were disappointing – but it's the folk who hide behind a mask that really push my buttons. Social media gives us a window into people's worlds, but it's a window covered in Vaseline into a carefully lit and curated room. Look behind the ring light and discover the piles of washing on the bedroom floor if you'd like a different story.

The irony is, I often mask myself. Sometimes I feel frightened, shy, burned and bruised. I ask you lots of questions that lure you into a sense of safety, when really I'm just controlling the conversation so you can't find out anything from me that might reveal a flaw or a weakness. It takes so much energy to curate a personality so carefully that it becomes like a second skin, a palatable social identity to match the photogenic angles on socials. To the outside world, everything is groovy. Even if you told me you could see right through the veneer, I would deny it and tell you to mind your own business, despite how much I desperately want to take you into my confidence and confess my hopes, fears, weirdness and fragility. I feel annoyed because, of course, you're the kind of person who would never judge me, and if I can't talk to you, then who can I confide in? Maybe I just don't know how trustworthy you are.

Masked people like me are everywhere, shielding themselves from pain and putting on a brave face. They might be one of your family members, but you probably won't know because you never really ask them anything about themselves, and even if you did they would give you a generic answer before changing the subject because they still haven't found the words to tell you just how awful you made them feel when they were at their most vulnerable. You might be friends with one of them, enjoying their company and generosity because they always make you feel good, lifted, supported and celebrated. You might be in a relationship with one, so afraid of losing you that they sometimes swallow their words if they're feeling hurt because they don't believe you'll ever forgive them if they put their selfish needs first. You might be sitting next to one of these people right now. You might be holding a book written by one of them. Hiding in plain sight. Right in front of your nose.

My identity is complex. As I swim up and down the slow lane of the pool, I wonder if I will get to a place where I feel safe enough to show my authentic self without fear of judgement. What will it take for me to be comfortable to do that? I think and swim, knowing with each lap I might get closer to that place. In here at least, I am in the right lane.

I score my identity as a 3 because I am generally comfortable with who I am, but I could feel more whole in this space. I would love to be able to feel more honest in more situations.

What is your score for identity?

. . . .

Why is it that number?

. . . .

. . . .

. . . .

. . . .

. . . .

What would you like to work on?

. . . .

. . . .

. . . .

. . . .

. . . .

2. INTIMACY

Close familiarity or friendship; cosy, private or relaxed

> "I've had huge issues my entire life around self-image, self-worth and guilt. I've had lots of therapy for it. I've been carrying shame since having conversion therapy when I was a teenager, and I hadn't realized that this wasn't my shame. This was shame that had been given to me."
>
> – PETER, 53

Between the ages of 18 and 30, the one place you would absolutely not find me was on a Club 18–30 holiday. Just the memory of the adverts makes my toes curl. Confident, boisterous, horny people, getting drunk, having lots of sex and making mischief and ... why is that such a bad thing? It sounds like the kind of holiday I'd love to go on now! But back then, I knew I wasn't welcome in those spaces anyway. They were for straight people only.

At school, in our final year, we had something called Activities Week. The jewel in the crown was called "Mediterranean Water Sports", a week-long adventure holiday full of swimming, scuba diving and snorkelling in the south of France. There was no way in hell I was going. Firstly, I was so ashamed of my body back then, the thought of spending a week in a Speedo was out of the question. Next were the thoughts of seeing all the hot boys in my year in their Speedos and having to sleep in a dormitory with them. Lastly, there was no way my parents could afford for me to go. Instead, I signed up for a week of activities at the school with the other losers where we watched lots of TV, interviewed our teachers and made a newsletter about all the activities in which we had taken part. I don't remember what the newsletter was called, but The Virgin Times would have been an appropriate title. All the hot, popular kids were in France. We knew our place. Kids in my school were sexually active from a young age. I remember being 13 and hearing my next-door neighbour, 13, having sex with his 13-year-old girlfriend. I lay on my bed listening to him grunting, wishing it was me instead of her. Boys and girls were always getting together and breaking up and getting drunk and being fingered and getting blow jobs. None of this was available to me. All the sexual experimenting going on was happening behind a locked laboratory door, and I did not have the key. I started to believe that pleasure, particularly sexual pleasure, was just not available to me. At the same time, AIDS was wiping out a generation of gay men who had only just started enjoying the freedom to fuck without consequence.

There was a window of time between decriminalizing homosexuality and AIDS when gay people could live their best sexy lives. It didn't last long. I grew up hearing about the "gay plague", and on some level, I believed that was my future. I thought that if anyone ever wanted to have sex with me, I'd end up dead. The law at that time meant that the age of consent for gay men was 21, so not only did I run the risk of death, I could also be arrested. Frankie Goes To Hollywood were banned by BBC Radio 1, a national UK radio station, for making a song about gay sex. It was a confusing time. Thankfully, I was such a mess then that nobody wanted to have sex with me anyway, so despite believing I was living a criminal life, I was at risk of neither incarceration nor Kaposi's sarcoma.

Even at university, I was a sexual disaster. The first time I was invited to share my friend's bed to sleep over after a late night out, not only did I leave my pants on, I kept my jeans on too. And a belt. He just laughed and said I was really sweet. He kissed my forehead and rolled over to sleep. I lay there awake all night, my hard-on squeezing against the zip of my jeans, wishing I could just ask him to hold me. I couldn't find the words.

I've been speaking with people about their relationships with their sexuality by asking them to imagine that they can pull their sexuality out of themselves and let it take on human form. I ask them to picture their sexuality saying, "Love, we need to go to couples' counselling." Then, I ask them, "What would your sexuality say to the therapist about your relationship with it?"

Mine would be sitting in a chair looking at me through half-closed eyes. Maybe smoking a fag and waggling a foot, with as much pent-up frustration as a cobra about to strike. I don't think it's very happy with me. It wants to shake me and shout "WHY?!" and maybe fall to its knees and weep. It looks at me, with compassion, and shakes its head.

"He is so afraid of me," it says to the therapist. "He doesn't seem to believe how good I am for him. He keeps locking me out. I wish he would just hold me, and stop being so scared of me."

It's true, despite PrEP, Doxy-PEP, sexual health clinics, sex education and "undetectable = untransmittable", I am still quite afraid to let my sexuality fully express itself. Carrie Fisher once wrote that she was so addicted to smoking, she would crave a cigarette while smoking one. Part of me thinks I'd be like that if I really gave in to my sexual urges, craving a man while fucking one.

I heard the word "promiscuous" a lot in relation to gay men when I was growing up. Straight people said they (we) hopped from bed to bed, shagging everything in sight, going to non-stop parties and orgies. At the same time, I also heard that gay men were incredibly lonely, sitting at home with their mothers, crying into their knitting because their lives were so sad. Who were these Schrödinger's Queers, both virgins and whores? In midlife, I can step back from all of the misinformation and fear, and try to make sense of it. I understand that pleasure is more than sex, but both are available. I fall firmly on the side of sex as an act of creation, not procreation, bringing joy and pleasure bursting into the world (or over someone's face). I realize now that the locked laboratory of pleasure never actually needed a key. I just had to smash in its back doors. My opportunity now is to experiment with ways of finding, experiencing and pursuing pleasure in as many ways I can, because it's okay to do that. I need to say that, and hear it, more often. I may be too old for Club 18–30, but I can visit The Lab any time. IYKYK. I just need to, as Frankie said, relax.

I score my intimacy as a 4 because my relationship to it is so much better than it used to be, but I have a lot further to go before I feel totally comfortable in expressing, owning and sharing my needs and feelings.

What's your score for intimacy?

. . . .

Why that number?

. . . .

. . . .

. . . .

. . . .

. . . .

. . . .

What would you like to work on?

. . . .

. . . .

. . . .

. . . .

. . . .

. . . .

3. MENTAL WELLBEING

A state of mind that allows us to function well and cope with life's challenges

> "I actually thought my parents would be alright. I thought I was overblowing the concern, but I was incorrect. Both of them took it really badly and made me swear I wouldn't tell anybody else. It's a whole drama."
>
> – LAYLA, 43

As a rule, I don't believe in burning books. It's a bit too right-wing for me. Just look at any dystopian novel: if it starts with book burnings, it usually ends in global destruction. The exception to my book-burning rule is what I call My Book of False Fairy Tales. One day, it will be ablaze, part of the poisoned library of stories people told me, about me, that no longer serve me.

Stories shape us. Stories can create and destroy us. Stories are grenades made of words. I've always loved the power in stories. Growing up, I spent a lot of time in the library, hiding from the hard kids at school who used to chase me down the street calling me a poof. Home wasn't much better. My mum was in the process of developing a chronic alcohol addiction, which made it hard for me to feel safe. Everything was unpredictable. The library was a peaceful, ordered sanctuary. Since I was a kid, around 1,000 public libraries in the UK have closed. All of those safe spaces, gone.

My parents separated just before I went to secondary school, but I never told anyone. Instead, I took the opportunity to tell stories to my new friends about how everything was just fine, everywhere, all the time. I never showed vulnerability or anything that might call attention to my difference. To this day, when someone asks me how I am, my knee-jerk reaction is to say, "I'm fine."

And on the whole, that's true. I am, mainly, fine. We are, mainly, fine. Little me back in the library could never have dreamed he would be here, telling this story, married, living in London ... that was not supposed to be my story.

Here are some of the stories I heard about me, about us, growing up:

- "You're going to die of AIDS." – The government
- "You're an unnatural pervert." – The church
- "We need to protect you from older, predatory gays." – Society
- " ..." – My dad

My mum, on the other hand, was a prolific storyteller, churning out such unique tales as:

- "Life is going to be so hard for you."
- "I'm not going to believe you're gay until it's confirmed by a psychiatrist."
- "What did I do to make you this way?"
- "You're so selfish for not giving me grandchildren."

All of these stories, even though none of them were true, made their way onto the shelves of my internal library. And I believed them. I used them as the ink to pen my own stories, in which I told myself:

- "I don't deserve happiness."
- "Nothing I do is ever going to be good enough."
- "People don't think I'm talented, they just feel sorry for me."

And, maybe even worse, I used them to write stories about others like me.

- "Those people prancing around at Pride are giving us a bad name."
- "Why would I want to sleep with him? He's so camp, I might as well sleep with a woman."
- "Ew, he goes to gay saunas – that's disgusting."

My internal library was once a toxic place. A library of lies, false fables and fake fairy tales. But in my 50s, I have some distance from the stories. I've even been able to believe that I can throw some of them away, to re-write the narrative. It helped when my mum died 18 years ago. She had been drinking herself to death all my adult life, and for years I worried I would follow her down that path, as if I had no choice. I eventually cracked and told my husband about my fears.

He smiled, held my hand and said, "But that's not your story. Your mum's story is not your story. It is hers, not yours. You get to write your own story." That simple truth liberated me. I had a choice in the story I told myself about my own future. I wonder what amount of liberation might be possible if I also separate the stories about my queerness into those that serve me and those that don't, a sort of internal library fumigation.

This is the story I wish I had been told growing up:

> You're gay? Brilliant. You're going to have a really interesting life filled with wonderful people.
>
> You get to decide how to express what it means to be you. You don't have to conform to any standards that don't apply to you. They're all made up anyway. You have a special kind of confidence inside you: a queer wholeness. You are not broken. You are whole, just as you are.
>
> The world will try to convince you that there's something wrong with you. There isn't.
>
> People will judge you for being yourself. The problem is them, not you.
>
> It's okay to be compassionate to those people. You might even forgive them. And it's okay if you feel really fucking angry, too. Anger is potential energy. You don't have to be nice, or fit in, or be accepted. You don't need anyone's approval except your own. You might decide to be a parent when you're older, but you don't have to feel any pressure there. It's okay to have kids, and okay to not. Legacy doesn't come in the form of children.

> Your difference gives you empathy. You'll see the world clearly, unable to ignore the cracks and contradictions. You can have one partner for life, or none, or as many as you like – sometimes at the same time. Anyone who makes a judgement on how you choose to express your sexuality is just projecting their own lack of imagination. Sexual pleasure is your right. Sex is the most natural, delicious, pure source of joy. There is no guilt or shame when it comes to your body.
>
> The people who tell you that your life is going to be difficult because you're gay will forget to tell you that they're the ones making it that way. You don't have to give yourself a hard time for falling over obstacles they put in your way. Just walk your own path. There is absolutely nothing wrong with being who you are. Being more of who you are is the only and best way to live.

The realization I can tell myself all of this now is like throwing open the windows of the poisoned library and clearing the fog. I'm learning to forgive myself for believing those stories.

There's something called the illusory truth effect, a psychological phenomenon where something is more likely to be perceived as true when it is continually repeated, regardless of whether it's a lie or not. The only thing I ever did wrong with my queerness was that I believed the lies people told about it. If we tell new stories, rewrite them, we can replace those fake fables with new, nourishing narratives.

In my 50s, the truth is that:

- My queerness is power.
- My queerness is community.
- My queerness is wholeness.
- My queerness is glorious.

It's time to shut down the poisoned library for good, to set the books on fire and watch those toxic narratives burn. Let's bask in the glow of its flames and warm each other. Throw our new story grenades made of good words, better words, and create new explosions of truthful, beautiful stories about who we really are, and what we can really be when we embrace our queer wholeness. The library is closed.

I score my mental wellbeing as a 2 because generally I feel whole and happy. I understand that happiness does not necessarily mean mental wellbeing, but it is a good indicator for me that I am heading in the right direction.

What do you score your mental wellbeing?

. . . .

Why that number?

. . . .

. . . .

. . . .

. . . .

. . . .

. . . .

What would you like to work on?

. . . .

. . . .

. . . .

. . . .

. . . .

. . . .

4. SELF-EXPRESSION

Differentiating from others through words and action our personality, feelings, thoughts and ideas

> "I'm going on a yoga retreat in January and it's all shared dorms. I realize I do have a little bit of a hangover of that fear, seeming predatory. If we're at dinner on the first night and I mention my girlfriend, is someone else in the dorm with me gonna be like, 'Oh, she's perving on me'?"
>
> – ABI, 43

I clicked on an advert for a hair transplant centre in Turkey because I was feeling nosey, and now Instagram can't stop forcing photos of middle-aged guys with thick, luscious locks in my face. Sadly, I think I'm already past the point of transplantation. My only decision now is toupee or not toupee. The answer to that question is, of course, no, I actually think a shaved head suits me.

As a teenager, I adored having, and abusing, hair. I went through enough hairspray to cause a Paul-shaped hole in the ozone layer, back-combing and setting my fringe into one solid mass. I bleached it blond, dyed it black and eventually shaved it off when my hair had decided enough was enough and gave up trying to grow. At the time, I thought it looked great, even in my Kurt Cobain, shoulder-length grease phase, but for some reason nobody told me it was terrible. Only years later did a friend confess that she didn't quite know what look I was going for, as the Nirvana hair was combined with way-too-orange make-up, my favourite lime green blazer, four earrings, one nose ring and one eyebrow ring. Confused chic. For someone who grew up wanting to be as invisible as possible, I had a knack for drawing attention to myself. My fashion in my 20s was standard: Docs and a Levi's denim jacket. My 30s were shirts and shoes. In my 40s, I started wearing bow ties, grew a beard and got more tattoos. In my 50s, I wouldn't necessarily say I am striking or particularly punk, but somehow I've managed to work out how to put a look together. Occasionally, Dan will shout "Mutton!" when I open a parcel from ASOS and he spies something with sequins.

It took several decades for the moment to come, but I am finally very happy with how I look. I smell good, thanks to a slightly more sophisticated choice of fragrance. I am tactile and a very good cuddler. I can't speak for anyone else on how I taste, but I hope it's satisfying. I am, sensorily, pretty content.

The part that needs work is my voice. Not how it sounds, because I quite like it, and people compliment me on it all the time, which is very kind. It's more about how I use it, or don't use it, as the case may be. I have become decidedly grumpy and vocal when walking in the street, tutting and swearing at people who stop at the top of an escalator. I am that pass-agg person who says "You're welcome" when I hold a door open for you and you don't say thanks. I sigh when people get on the Tube without letting me off, and when someone is nose-deep in their phone and about to walk into me, I say, "Look up, for fuck's sake."

I'm a vocal menace in the streets, but sadly, I'm not so verbal in the sheets. I find it hard to express what I want and need sexually. I can't seem to find the words for it, so I usually stay quiet. A friend once told me that sex should never be silent, that we should release sounds and moans like animals, giving in to our pre-verbal urges. I struggle with that. When I was pre-teen, I would sometimes hear my parents having sex in their bedroom. I'd be downstairs watching *Saturday Superstore*, and I'd hear the bed squeaking above, or the occasional gasp. It made me feel quite sick. Channelling my inner pensioner, I would tut and turn the volume up on the TV, muttering about how disrespectful it was for them to do that. I felt somehow guilty for being in the house, as if I had any other choice.

Despite only being in their 20s, my parents had quite a reserved attitude to sex and their bodies. I don't remember ever seeing either of them naked. The bathroom door was locked when occupied. Towels and dressing gowns were always worn after baths, and sex was never discussed. When something slightly raunchy came on TV, they changed the channel. They never spoke to me about sex as I was growing up, leaving any kind of "education" to school. When I came home, the day we watched a baby being born on *Living and Growing*, my mum hugged me and said, "Now you know how it all happens." There was a conspiracy of silence when it came to chatting about carnal issues. I'm sure that contributed to my feelings of disgust when I would hear them fucking. How dare they bring that kind of behaviour into our house? I never spoke about it to them, though, as I was also bound to silence in the conspiracy. It meant I was never spoken to about sexual health and definitely not sexual pleasure, even from a straight perspective. I had to work it out for myself, carrying a small stone of sexual sickness in my stomach at all times.

It still stumps me when someone asks, "What are you into?" I honestly don't know. Or if I do know, I'm very reserved and uncomfortable to talk about it. I'm fine with the behaviour, just not so good when it comes to asking for what I want or need. Perhaps it doesn't help that I rebel against the trend to label myself a top or a bottom, a dom or a sub, a this or a that. Why can't we be all those things, or none of them, or something else? Paradoxically, my lack of language when it comes to sex is the opposite of my imagination that can pretty much conjure up any scenario and work with it. I have no idea how many men I have had sex with. I stopped counting in my 20s. When I see online quizzes aimed at straight people, in which five partners or more is counted as very liberal and experienced, I realize that those scales are not for me.

I don't have an issue with quantity, or even quality, of sex. It's one of conversation. I don't have many friendships where I can talk about the sex I'm having, or not. There is still a hesitancy in me to talk about being in a 26-year committed relationship that is also open. I believe, truly, that the opinions of other people about my relationship are totally irrelevant to me, yet there are long-term, deep friendships where "don't ask, don't tell" applies. There is a part of my wholeness that stays very hidden because I don't know how to express myself in words, which is ironic for a writer. I think I'm good at sex, and I enjoy it, but I am silent when it comes to talking about my participation in it, maybe the way I wished my parents had been more silent with their sex life. Maybe I think I'll make others feel a little sick if they hear me talk about having sex.

I was never affected by slut-shaming, or as it was called when us midlifers were younger, "promiscuity"; but on some level, I decided to go against Salt-N-Pepa's wisdom, making my mantra, "Let's *not* talk about sex, baby." Unless I do something about it, there will be a part of me that remains locked away from the world.

Straight people don't seem to care about that. When the woman in accounts announces that she and Brian are expecting a baby, I can't help but picture them fucking. Straight sex is represented everywhere, in every TV show, book, film, coffee advert, sports car and skyscraper. It is literally rammed down our throats. I wonder if a lifetime of choking on straight sex has affected my vocal cords? At school, my friend Diane had a theory that everything came down to sex. We had to study to pass exams to get a job to make money to attract someone to have sex with. The answer to everything was sex.

So, when I see those Instagram adverts for hair transplants, I hear Diane's voice in my head. It's all about sex. Do the people who get hair plugs do it just for themselves, or because they think it will get them more sex? When I was cosplaying an orange Kurt Cobain, it had the opposite effect on people. They were confused, unclear and unattracted because they found me confusing, unclear and unattractive. In my 50s, I feel so much more attractive and much clearer about who I am. I just need to work on the part of me that is still confused about the language to use when it comes to expressing myself sexually.

When I see friends or followers getting throuple-d up, or declaring themselves poly, or spending weekends at intimacy retreats and in cuddle puddles, I feel envious of their freedom to express that part of themselves. I have no desire to be in a throuple – one husband is quite enough – but I desire to be able to talk about desire with a heavy, blue-balled passion that seems to be on the permanent edge of explosion.

As I said at the beginning of this book, people keep telling me, "You write the book you need to read." Self-expression takes many forms: clothes, hair, tattoos, books, music, piercings, food, politics and sex. It's time for an exorcism, to let go of the chains that have held me back, possibly to find new chains that can move me forward. This needs further conversation, and good examples of those start with a great question. So, I ask: what might be possible if I were to find the words to talk about my sexuality in a way that honours the brilliance of queer sex? Celebrates it. Talks it up. Liberates it. What if I could express myself instead of repressing myself?

Despite all this, I score my self-expression as a 3. It might be the place I feel most whole despite the challenges I have faced and created for myself. It's not quite complete, but it's something that I can lean on when I feel less whole in other areas.

What do you score your self-expression?

. . . .

Why that number?

. . . .

. . . .

. . . .

. . . .

What would you like to work on?

. . . .

. . . .

. . . .

. . . .

5. SELF-ACCEPTANCE

Owning and embracing who you are without exception

> We'd be watching TV, and my Grandma would call certain men 'gaylords' and say it was disgusting behaviour and it wasn't natural."
>
> – GORDON, 47

I found a pair of underpants in the gym shower, and my whole life flashed in front of my eyes. Well, "finding" sounds too deliberate, like I was looking for them. The pants were just there in the shower cubicle I happened to go into.

My gym is in the City (London's main financial district), so I'm usually surrounded by bankers, brokers and insurers, but on Pants Day – as I now think of it – the changing room was empty, apart from me. There are 12 shower cubicles in the changing room, and of all the showers in all the gyms in all the world, I walked into the one with a pair of pants hanging there. It made my stomach churn.

Changing rooms have always been an uncomfortable place for me. At secondary school, I became incredibly self-conscious in a way that my straight classmates seemed never to experience. Those boys would whip each other's bums with wet towels and hang shirts from the end of their hard-ons. Cocks were commented on and laughed at. I didn't dare look at them, in case my body gave me away.

In the 1980s, coming out at school was not an option. So, I stared at the floor and pretended it wasn't happening, locking myself out of the boys' banter. It was a confusing space. It was apparently okay for them to point at someone's dick and call him "maggot" for the next four years, but if I looked at someone's dick for four milliseconds, I was called a poof. A pervert. Accused of having AIDS. All my dreams of men and love and sex got buried deep down where nobody could find them, locked away in a hidden hall of shame.

Straight boys, ironically, seem to be at their most boisterous when they're naked together. Not much has changed since 1985. In the gym last month, I heard one (straight) guy say to another, "Fucking hell, bro, your ass is really hairy," to which the bro replied, "Well, at least my cock doesn't look like a sausage roll." I was dying to look at sausage-roll-cock man, or Gregg as I called him, but the churning feeling of shame appeared in my stomach, and I turned away.

Anyway, back to Pants Day.

I stood in the shower cubicle looking at the abandoned pants, feeling curious. They were black briefs, size medium, from a brand called Swiss Adventurer. They appeared to be dry, but I had no idea how long they'd been hanging there. I did not dare touch them to find out if they were warm, although I was tempted.

Actually, I was tempted to do so much more than just touch them. I wanted to smell them, put them in my mouth, rub them over me. I didn't do any of those things because the acid in my stomach told me I must be some kind of pervert. Instead, I moved my head around the pants, trying to understand them.

No name label stitched in the back. They seemed clean. I had never heard of Swiss Adventurer before. They sounded exotic. Outdoorsy. Maybe the person who owned them was a hiker? Size medium meant he wasn't a tiny twink, but maybe more of a beefy, rugby-playing type. I pictured him meaty but solid.

I stood paralysed in that cubicle, wondering how many days or hours had passed since the pants had been forgotten there. What if it was only a few minutes earlier? What would happen if the Swiss Adventurer had left the gym, taken a few steps and thought, Shit, I don't remember putting me pants in my bag, before turning round, back into the gym. He would pass reception, making a pffft, what-a-twat gesture. He would get to the shower, but there'd be someone in there. He would push the door open, which would smack into my naked ass, and the first thing he'd see would be his pants stuffed in my mouth.

Back in reality, I needed to get out of the cubicle. I knew I should move to the one next door, which hopefully didn't contain any pants. But I thought to myself, Why should I move? I didn't deliberately choose the one with pants in it. It wasn't my fault. And why couldn't I just shower and pretend they weren't hanging there? In fact, I thought, I should just pick them up and, without sniffing them, throw them over the divider into the stall next door. I'd have to touch them, though, and, of course, that would be the moment when the owner would walk in.

I decided that the easiest and most sensible thing to do would be to put my towel back on and move to the next cubicle. I took one last look at the pants and left. The cubicle next door was thankfully empty, but even as I showered, the pants mocked me. "Coward." "Pervert." "Queer." I left the showers with the image of the pants seared into my brain.

The changing room was still empty. No sign of anyone. I dressed quickly and left the gym, wondering how Eric the cleaner might deal with the situation. Would he even give it a second thought to throw the pants in the bin? Would he feel shame? Shame whispers that I am in the wrong for being in the same space as a pair of forgotten pants. That someone would think I had intentionally put myself in there or had been lurking in the changing rooms, waiting for someone to forget their underwear so I could stuff them in my mouth.

The voice of shame is old. It has been there for a long time, in my stomach. My metabolism is slow when it comes to breaking down and expunging my shame. I wonder, how can we boost our shame metabolism? How can we convert it into energy? The performance artist Marina Abramovic says, "Do things with your shame. Expose yourself in a shameless way. It's very important to be vulnerable and to show the things you're afraid and ashamed of to everybody – not just to people you love, but also to the public."

So, to speed up my shame metabolism, I want to quickly mention other moments from my Hall of Shame. They include how ashamed I was of being bullied at school, of being chased along the street and being threatened every day. I was ashamed of the time our phone bill arrived and my mum had to sit down because it was so high, thanks to my addiction to premium-rate telephone sex lines where I listened to men pretending to fuck each other for 50 pence per minute. I was ashamed of my parents finding out I was gay at 15 when they read my diary and discovered my fantasy of having a threesome with George Michael and Morten Harket from a-ha. I was ashamed of the moment I thought maybe I could put my dick in the end of the hoover, and so I did. Would not recommend. Those scars are hard to explain.

I feel lighter for saying all that. Less ashamed. A little embarrassed, but I can deal with that. Shame and embarrassment are close cousins, but where embarrassment is fleeting and felt on the face, shame is old and inside. Embarrassment is the time I went to a Halloween fancy dress party in head-to-toe green body paint dressed as The Incredible Hulk. It turned out it was a Halloween dinner party, and not only was I the only person dressed up, the first guest to see me said, "Ahhh, Shrek!" Embarrassment makes a good story. There is nothing good about shame.

There's a gift that comes with middle age: the gift of reflection and introspection, picking through the fragments that wounded us growing up, inspecting them and letting them go. Sharing our stories without fear, or care, or judgement. Holding them up to the light and watching those that no longer serve us come out of the shadows and disappear.

I score my self-acceptance as a 3 because it feels like I am finally able to believe in myself at this stage of my life, but I want it to be much more integrated. Unshakeable. There is more to be done here.

What do you score your self-acceptance?

. . . .

Why that number?

. . . .

. . . .

. . . .

. . . .

What would you like to work on?

. . . .

. . . .

. . . .

. . . .

6. BELONGING

Affinity for, ownership of or membership to a place or situation

"In chosen family, someone is saying, 'We're not related in any way, but I'm here for you. I will fight battles by your side. I will die on that hill for you. I am here no matter what, and I'm choosing to do that.' When people say blood is thicker than water and all that rubbish, no – when it comes to chosen family, the fact that we choose to put ourselves out there, I think it's beautiful, it's powerful, and it's a source of strength."

– EVA, 44

As a child, nobody gave me any rules about growing up as a well-adjusted gay person, so I adopted the ones I saw from family, neighbours or TV. Straight people, it appeared, had simple, well-established guidelines for what it meant to belong to society. A social scaffolding they could lean into and build themselves against: grow up, leave school, get a job, get married, have kids, get promoted, have grandchildren, retire, die. If you followed that framework, you were generally going to fit in. You couldn't do anything too weird, like vote Green or wear pink if you're a man; if you didn't, then you'd probably be okay. It turned out that the expectations and norms of society didn't apply to me but I still tried to force myself into them, like Cinderella's big, handsome sister shoving my foot into her glass slipper. It did not fit, and it hurt, but I kept it on anyway.

I have to preface this whole story by saying that from the age of 1 to 35, I was a fucking hot-mess disaster, probably because I was mentally hobbling around, in pain, unable to breathe. I kept trying to conform, but my real self kept bursting out of the edges. At 17, I moved to London, hoping to feel a little looser. My first proper job was in the office of a homecare agency. I wore orange shirts with purple waistcoats – by choice – and used a messenger bag with a picture of Homer Simpson saying "d'oh!" on it. It was a small, family-run company that had no interest in how people dressed for work, until we were sold to a global corporation. I got a new boss who told me I needed to sharpen up, lose the Simpsons bag and get a proper suit. She told me her motto was "FIFO" – "fit in or fuck off".

She wasn't the only one who lived by that motto, although I didn't expect to find it hanging over Heaven (not the religious one, but the London LGBTQ+ nightclub). The first time I went was when I was about to turn 18. It was a group outing organized by one of the more experienced elders of my friend group, Jonny, who was 20. He told us that getting into Heaven was really strict, and they might ask us to prove we were gay. I never questioned that he was joking, instead imagining the kinds of things I might have to do to the bouncers to get in. Sadly, they waved me straight through.

I spent the night entranced, seeing hot bodies, sweaty torsos and furious snogging everywhere. For a boy who had just left Scotland, the club lived up to its name. I was, indeed, in heaven. I thought I was finally with my people. I belonged. I never actually snogged or went home with anyone from Heaven. People paid me little attention, as I didn't meet the ripped-body standards of the 1991 scene, so although I was allowed entry, I was never fully invited to participate. I didn't completely fit in. It was "fit in or fuck off" – with a silent "fuck off".

The queer community didn't feel as welcoming as I thought it would. During an interview for this book, someone said something that made me laugh. We were talking about our relationship with the community, and he said, "I'm not one of those apex gays, you know, the ones in their Speedos on the cruise ship. I'm at the other end of the spectrum." That sentence is so loaded with meaning, so heavy with feeling, so perfect. I knew exactly who he was talking about, and I got a sense of where they existed on his social hierarchy. I loved that he called it a spectrum, as it meant there was an opposite space where he thought he lived. He told me, "The other end of the spectrum is me. I'm a middle-aged single gay man with no gay friends who spends his time going to dinner with straight couples."

Et voilà, a community continuum was born: from single gay person with no gay friends to gays in Speedos on a boat. I began asking others where they would place themselves on that scale, and an incredible amount of nuance emerged. Pretty much everyone could locate themselves somewhere. Mostly, us midlife queers are an indoor bunch who like peace and quiet, with the occasional trip to a nightclub on a bank holiday weekend, but more likely an outing to a flower market because we get up early these days. Who needs an alarm clock with my bladder? Bars are too noisy to hear each other, and isn't it nicer to just be at home and in bed by 10pm anyway? Actually, that's just me. There were, of course, plenty of folk who still have stamina, and I salute their refusal to stop dancing. My favourite reaction to this spectrum was the non-binary artist who said, "I'm queer, fuck your continuum. I walk around it in a circle flicking the Vs to gay conformity."

Our relationship to the queer community changes over time, just as relationships naturally change among families and friends, with many of us feeling more on the margins of each as time goes by. I've had a lot of conversations that ended with: "I'm not sure where I belong anymore." Apps like Grindr or SCRUFF try to fix it with a simple solution. Put yourself into a box. Twink. Jock. Top. Bottom. Kink. Poly. While it's true that bears of a feather fuck together, isn't it also nice to enjoy all the flavours of the rainbow? Sameness is soothing, but difference is life.

Society itself seems to be on an eternal quest to make us unbelong. To separate us, divide us and conquer us. And it's not just straight people. I remember the days when things were much simpler. Straight people = bad. Gay people = good. We could have nice, easy them-versus-us arguments about how awful they were while they told us how wrong we were. I am all in favour of being with people like me, who feel easy to be with. Similarity can be incredibly safe, but it can lead to apathy and lazy agreement. We're in a different era now, an era of community complexity. We have, rightly, acknowledged that the LGBTQ+ community contains universes of difference. Unfortunately, our galaxy also contains some hostile aliens. They look and sound like us, but they're very different under the skin.

These people include the awful LGB Alliance UK and their hostile, unnecessary war on trans people. Gays on apps who still say no fats, no fems, no Asians. Bears snubbing twinks. People who kink-shame or show hostility to those in open relationships. Those who mock queer folk who seek monogamy. It's a lot. Sometimes it feels like the fastest growing threat to queer people is queer people. I tell myself that maybe these conflicts are just the growing pains of a maturing community entering its rebellious teenage phase, but it's happening in a cultural climate of emboldened hostility toward us, where empathy is a scarce resource. It means, for me, I have a really confused set of answers to the question of belonging. Several of my long-held heroes have toppled from their pedestals. The call is coming from inside the Haus.

As the emerging elders of the community, we have to stand up for those of us who are under attack. When I was growing up, people used to say gays should be shipped off and put on an island. Back then, I was outraged, but I quite like the idea of that now, especially if they pay for the flights. How wonderful to live on this paradise island, a place based on understanding, curiosity, compassion and joy. A place where we celebrate each other. A place where we can truly belong.

Actually, we don't need to go anywhere to make that a reality. We just have to be less cunty to each other. Kinder. More curious. Show each other our soft underbellies, letting our vulnerability out to play. Community without conformity. The queer community is not something that happens "over there". It's here. It's me. It's everything I say and do. It's like when you're running late to get somewhere and you're stuck in traffic, so you call and say, "Arrrrghhh, sorry it's not my fault I'm stuck in traffic," but you're not in traffic, you are the traffic. The person behind is blaming you. And someone is blaming them.

So, if we are the community, all of the time, it's up to us to make it a better place. Only now in my 50s am I starting to understand that I really only need to belong to myself and my husband. To belong means to fit in. To be in the right place. Dan and I fit. We are each other's right place. But I want more than that. I want to be part of something bigger as well. Living unapologetically as myself in the safety of a relationship is great, but what if Dan gets sick or dies? Where will I belong in the absence of my tether? I have no desire to integrate back into straight society. It's up to me to create the spaces in which I wish to belong.

Belonging anywhere means not belonging everywhere. A friend recently asked if I realized I was sounding quite radical these days. "Heterophobic," he said. I think I'm just tired. Tired of having to worry if I'm going to get punched for holding my husband's hand in the street. Tired of reading transphobic articles in the press every single day. Tired of conversations that start with "Don't you think diversity has gone too far?", as came up at a recent family dinner.

Unlike Cinderella, I don't aspire to live happily ever after. I'd be good with content from now on. I want to pick up the pen in the middle of the story and write the ending that suits me, not anyone else. Getting older has given me the strength to be able to finally say, "Fit in? Fuck off." I score my belonging as both a 1 and a 5. This one is complicated for me because I realize it's pretty contextual. In the right places, I feel utterly at home. In less hospitable spaces, I have a distinct sense of being the alien in the room. I'm fascinated by how wildly my score shifts on this one – there's definitely further exploration needed.

What do you score your belonging?

. . . .

Why that number?

. . . .

. . . .

. . . .

. . . .

What would you like to work on?

. . . .

. . . .

. . . .

. . . .

. . . .

7. LIFE TRANSITIONS

Significant newness leading to change, growth or adaptation

> "The only thing I wish is that I had been more radical earlier and cut my parents out sooner, more substantially and quicker."
>
> – LIOR, 45

There's been a distinct shift in my Grindr messages since turning 50: less "show hole" and more "hey, Daddy". I don't mind. I wish when I was younger, I'd been able to contact handsome, successful, funny writers, instead of relying on the men's underwear pages of the Freeman's catalogue for my entire sex life.

Instagram ads, however, are less "hey, Daddy" and more "choke me, Daddy", in that they go straight for the throat. "Have you planned your funeral?" asks one grey-haired man. "Problems with erections?" says a happy young woman. Recently, I got an ad that asked, "Do you get a sweaty back?", and when I ignored it, they came back twice as hard with "Do you suffer from swamp ass?" Thing is, no, I haven't planned my funeral. Sometimes, I do get trouble with erections, and in certain situations, my ass can get – there's no other word for it – swampy. That's the trouble with algorithms. They know us too well. It's not all bad, though. I clicked on an ad for over-50s home insurance, and we saved 20 per cent on our annual policy. I have a confusing relationship with getting older. On the one hand, it's an opportunity to thrive and live the way I want to, and yet it's feeling more real that there's less road ahead than behind. I don't think I'm having a midlife crisis, certainly not the red-Ferrari kind. Maybe it's more of an existential crisis. At least it's cheaper and doesn't involve hanging out at strip clubs.

More often than before, though, I wonder if I'm living a meaningful life. It's a big question. The philosopher Søren Kierkegaard said we should each find a truth that is personally meaningful and worth living and dying for. Finding a truth implies the existence of that truth, and maybe that's my problem: I've either never had one, or I've misplaced it. Maybe it fell behind the sofa. I believed so many lies about myself growing up that it's sometimes difficult to find the truth.

Turning 50 also meant nice gifts. My friend Jonas bought me a poster made up of 4,000 empty circles. Four thousand dots, representing the numbers of weeks an average person lives. Four thousand weeks. Jonas used my date of birth when he ordered it, so it arrived pre-filled, with more than half the dots already blacked out. According to the poster I've been alive for 2,615 weeks, and I have 1,385 to go.

Strangely, I haven't filled in any of the dots since I got the poster. Am I in denial? It all feels very linear, like the world's easiest maze where you start at dot 1 and end at dot 4,000. Within the deceptively simple journey lies an impossible maze of meaning. What are we supposed to do with all those dots? How are we supposed to make meaning from our lives? Judith Butler says, "We find meaning through the expression of our authentic selves," but that's hard. Those of us queer folk now in middle age grew up not in the shadow of oppression, but staring at the bright, blazing glare of it, burning spots on our vision forever. We were told from an early age that it wasn't okay to be our authentic selves. Life was not easy. When I look again at the 4,000 dots on the poster, I wonder how many of the 2,615 filled-in dots were spent being able to live truly, openly and authentically as myself? This stage of life offers us an opportunity to pause, reflect and think about how we might live more deliberately for the rest of our days. We haven't come this far, through all of that, to accept mediocrity now.

Existentially speaking, there is a positive to that. The philosopher William James thought that those of us who have gone through intense suffering, who seek deeper meaning, will ultimately be happier. The "twice born", he calls us. Maybe our middle age is our second coming (out). We need to celebrate our second coming out!

A common theme of the people who I spoke to when shaping this book was one of reaching this age and feeling stuck. We didn't have maps on how to get here, so we forged our own paths. We threw ourselves into work, sex, drugs – perhaps all the above – and maybe we've reached a point where we just feel a bit out of place. How did we get here? What is "here" like? What happens next? How do we locate ourselves as middle-aged queer people in a straight world?

Midlife itself is full of contradictions. There's the irony of getting into peak confidence just around the time you start to need afternoon naps. In my case, the unhappiness I felt with my body throughout my 20s has been replaced by a celebratory sense of my sexiness, but my clubbing days are few and far between. A friend invited me to an event that started at 10 o'clock. "PM?" I asked. No thanks. Many philosophers say that finding meaning in life comes down to one question: do I have a purpose? I think that's a bit limiting, just to have one. It's a bit straight. Meaning doesn't have to be singular. It doesn't have to be linear. Why be so constrained by having a singular, life-defining purpose? Let's queer it up and have as many as we like.

Why not ask, "What are my purposes?"

Between now and the end of this impossible maze of meaning, I want to find ways to flourish through middle age and beyond. From midlife crisis to midlife confidence. Less existential and more experimental. So, with each of the passing dots approaching my allotted 4,000, I may not be asked so much to "show hole", but I will be showing my wholeness to everyone, whether they like it or not, until I have no dots left to give.

I score my life transitions as a 3 because I feel connected to my wholeness, knowing what has happened during the years it took me to reach middle age, and I am still here. I want to do more work on this area because the transitions that are coming feel more significant. Uncharted. I want to build some deeper connections to this that might fortify me for an unknown future.

What do you score your life transitions?

. . . .

Why that number?

. . . .

. . . .

. . . .

. . . .

. . . .

What would you like to work on?

. . . .

. . . .

. . . .

. . . .

. . . .

. . . .

8. LEGACY

Lasting impact of events and actions during a person's life

"It ends with me. This cycle ends with me. I am the most senior, oldest soul of this lineage, and my responsibility is to heal that of mine and the lives before me."

– NICHOLAS, 45

Three months after turning 50, I got chickenpox. I think it was part of my body's attempt to regain my youth. The week before being diagnosed, I felt lousy – tired, achy, grizzly, like a really bad cold was about to hit, but never quite broke through. The day before being diagnosed, I collapsed in the bathroom, and my husband found me on the floor, unresponsive. I came round quite quickly and found myself lying under the sink with no idea of how I got there. As I tried to make sense of it in my head, I thought, "Oh, maybe I'm dying." I'm embarrassed to admit that my first regret was not that I hadn't spent enough time with my family, but "Fuck, I didn't get to see my book published." Anyway, it turned out it was chickenpox that had made my body crash and reboot itself, and within a couple of weeks, everything was back to normal, except it was the first time I had ever contemplated that this might be the moment I die. It made me ponder my mortality, and also my legacy.

I could trace my family tree back to the dawn of time if I had the capacity, technology and resources needed for such a task. Hundreds of thousands of people who passed their genes around, handing down the inability to grow more than five-and-a-half feet tall, to exist with no hair on our heads but enough on our bums to see us through several cold winters. Each of my ancestors who survived sabre-toothed tiger attacks or poisoned berries that seemed like a good idea at the time gave something of themselves in my creation, and for that I am grateful. Also guilt-ridden. I have a lot of guilt about being the last of my name.

Growing up with the full awareness of my queerness, I realized from a young age that I was never going to have children. Of course, some queer people do have children, and in the 2020s, it's much more toward the acceptable end of the social continuum than when I was a kid. For the first 19 years of my life, though, it wasn't legal for gay couples to adopt children, and without that option I planned my future to be child-free. When I came out, one of my mum's many reactions was to cry and tell me I was selfish for denying her grandchildren. Ever the rationalist, I said, "But what if I was straight and infertile?", to which she replied, "At least you'd have tried."

The guilt that came with ending the family line sat heavy with me for a long time. Was I a waste of genes? Did all the effort of all those people in the history of my ancestry really end with this? With me? In some ways, it made me incredibly diligent. Some might call me an overachiever, while others would say I'm a try-hard. I don't think I was naturally clever or gifted in anything, but somehow, I was the first in my family to go to university. There's a part of me that is incredibly compelled to do something good with my life, to not waste the gifts my ancestors bestowed upon me.

Equally strong is the urge to do nothing, to leave no trace and eventually be forgotten. As I reminded my parents several times, I didn't ask to be born, so why should I bear any responsibility for anyone else's expectations on me? I did not apply for this position. On the days I spend bingeing *Taskmaster* – which Dan calls my straight guilty pleasure – or playing hours of pointless games on my phone, I achieve absolutely nothing. Is that okay? To achieve nothing? What about the stuff I've already achieved? At what point can I say, "That's enough"?

Legacy is more and more on my mind as I get older. It's a mental minefield that I navigate daily. Just when I think I'm okay with watching a third episode of *Baby Reindeer*, my brain explodes, hurling me in the air with the question "Why have you not written anything this good? You are wasting your life and becoming a massive failure!" Ultimately, that's the core of every mental minefield: the idea that I'm a failure. That, somehow, I've failed at life because I didn't pass on my genes and continue the human race. To be fair, I have distributed plenty of DNA and there are a lot of people who, if their bits had been different, might have got pregnant. See, Mum, I have been trying.

My relationship with failure is complicated. I've have recurring dreams where I turn up to the start line of the London Marathon wearing black leather shoes, or arrive at the job interview a day late, or get on the wrong bus, which means I miss the plane that was taking me to my dream home I just won on the lottery and now can't claim. I am not comfortable with failure. So, to counter this I have decided that I have already won at life. Nobody can take away everything I have already achieved, whether it's my degrees, or my 26-year relationship, or someone messaging me to say that I helped them with a problem. They all count. Whatever happens from now on, that's icing on the cake of success.

Every single one of us will be forgotten at some point. History is short and the future is infinite. Have as many children as you like, their ancestors will one day forget your name. Write as many books as you want, they'll all turn to dust eventually. But never stop trying. Never stop changing. I want to die as a person I don't yet know, someone unrecognizable to his younger self. My legacy is that I have survived as a queer person in this world for more than 50 years, and I fucking love it. My legacy is that my queerness is glorious. My legacy is that I will live purposefully, vividly and loudly queer for the rest of my days.

I am a middle-aged gay man who survived school, homophobic bullying, the AIDS crisis, several conservative governments, periods of depression and anxiety, and the biggest near-death experience of my life: chickenpox. I have not come this far to stop here.

I will not, and cannot, stop chasing what fuels me: the wish for every queer person on the planet to be able to live freely, without fear, as constantly evolving versions of themselves, understanding that they are magical, superpowered, wise, amazing, bright beacons of light in a beige and boring world full of straight people. That is our legacy. Is the desire for legacy just an ego-driven urge to prove that somehow we matter? Would it matter if we didn't matter? Does it mean we have to matter to everyone equally, or is it okay to just matter to a handful of people who would lose something if we were no longer in the world?

On a flight recently I sat next to a wonderful woman, and we got to chatting about life. In the space of under four hours, I learned that she runs a dog-grooming business, has one 17-year-old daughter, three failed relationships and a total disregard for her own self-care. She also shares a birthday with Madonna. As solo travellers on this occasion, we were both a little giddy about taking time out for ourselves. She had never been away on her own. Her daughter persuaded her to make space and focus on herself for a change. My book came up in conversation, as it does whenever I talk to anyone, and she was genuinely interested in the experiences of people who grew up queer. She told me that she had recently asked her daughter if she was doing okay, and if she was feeling comfortable with who she was and her sexuality, and how she was expressing it. How beautiful to be parented with such grace. She said she just wanted to make sure her daughter knew she could be whoever she was. That is legacy. I will carry that story with me wherever I go, knowing that for a brief moment, I was able to be in the company of someone who is the kind of parent I needed.

In a way, children are an easy legacy, which I say as a non-parent who has no idea what I am talking about when it comes to children. Of course it's not easy being a parent. To me, it seems like most people – straight people – see their children as their greatest, and sometimes only, achievement. Queer people have to make more of a deliberate and often convoluted route to parenthood, which I hope makes us even better at raising small people who feel totally loved. For me, I have chosen creation instead of procreation. It just never quite feels enough.

Perhaps legacy only comes when we let go of that attachment. To free ourselves of any need or desire to be anything or anyone other than who we are right now in this moment, creating and recreating a future for ourselves that has innumerable possibilities even if the one we choose is eating a tub of Ben & Jerry's in front of another episode of *Star Trek Voyager*. It is my life. I will do with it exactly what I wish. I may not write *Baby Reindeer*, but that's okay. Someone else already did. My work is to create something new and original, uniquely me. Living as a queer person in the singular expression of my purest, most deliberate self is my contribution to the ongoing urge to enter oblivion.

I score my legacy as a 4 because some days it haunts me and others I could not care less. There's obviously something there that needs to be explored. Maybe the fact I never believed I would make it this far has led me to feel confused about now having to even think about legacy. I want to do more on this.

What do you score your legacy?

. . . .

Why that number?

. . . .

. . . .

. . . .

. . . .

. . . .

What would you like to work on?

. . . .

. . . .

. . . .

. . . .

. . . .

. . . .

9. MORTALITY

Existing in the state of being destined to die

> "I want some of my ashes scattered on the floor of the Royal Vauxhall Tavern and some on Old Compton Street. I'm happiest surrounded by people who are happy to be themselves."
>
> – GARVIN, 57

My mum died when I was 35, which at the time felt pretty average but now seems young to lose a parent. People lose family at all times of their lives, so my experience is not unique, but it felt very ... specific.

On the day of her funeral, I was shocked that the whole world didn't just stop for a day to pay respects. After the formalities, I noticed that, for the first time in my life, I felt properly grown up. I had lost a parent. That's huge.

Since her death, I have discovered a new sense of life in myself. My most enjoyable, productive and creative times have happened since she died. I did some really good work and made a mark in my professional field of practice. I ran seven marathons. I did a doctorate. I started my own business. I wrote a book. Maybe those things would always have happened when I hit middle age, but I doubt they would if my mum had still been around. Her alcoholism was a shadow that blocked the sun, making my growth harder than it should have been. Today, I have much more compassion for her. I miss her now more than ever, but I'm glad she's no longer here going through the torment that she did, causing chaos in her wake. I hope she is at peace now. I am.

I don't think my mum would have liked being old. I'm almost at the age she was when she died, and while I feel in a good place, she certainly wasn't. She would be 70 if she were still alive, and I can imagine the horror that would evoke in her. She was vivid, vibrant and full of life. Old age would not have suited her. For me, though, I am enjoying the unfolding possibilities that getting older brings. The care-less-live-more era suits me. I hope it lasts.

My encounter with chickenpox was the nearest I've come to a near-death experience, and it was really nothing of the sort. Despite the relative ease of my recovery, I laid on the sofa, unsettled. I started to cry, feeling a confused mix of anger, frustration, fear and powerlessness. Dan started to cry, too, saying how afraid he had been that he was losing me. It was the closest I'd ever been to the boundary of my mortality. It was the first time in my life (other than after a few too many strawberry ciders) that I had experienced a total loss of control of my body and been helpless in the care of strangers. The story in hindsight is really un-dramatic. I had chickenpox, I fainted, I recovered. However, one of the consultants did make assumptions about me that almost derailed the diagnosis because I was married to a man, steering the conversation toward Monkey instead of Chicken where the pox was concerned.

There are much more harrowing stories than mine, of awful treatment by healthcare providers. Take the lesbian couple who miscarried a child after years of IVF, just for the consultant to say, "Well, you can just try again can't you?" Or the gay couple who had a child through surrogacy, who were stopped at the door by a hospital safeguarding officer who refused to let them leave with their daughter and made an emergency call to the child-protection team. Then there's the man whose husband had long-term, undiagnosed HIV and developed brain impairment, leading to admission to a nursing home, where the staff referred to him as "his friend" and eventually refused to let him wash his dead husband's body. People tell me that they worry about becoming ill and not being able to look after themselves; they also have a fear of having to engage with what is perceived, and often experienced, as a heteronormative, uninformed, discriminatory health and care system.

Middle age is a period when our mortality feels less like a shadow and more of a solid presence, maybe on the edge of our vision but firmly in the room. As I've said before, our generation is the first to be able to live openly, authentically as ourselves. Those who came before us were sometimes imprisoned, fired, arrested and attacked, and many of them were wiped out from AIDS. So, us midlifers have very few people to look to who have been able to tackle the issues that we're about to meet head-on.

Straight people will not solve this for us. We are all we have, and I hope we are enough. There is a tidal wave of middle-aged queer folk who will, sooner than we think, be using a lot of resources. Are our systems ready for us? Are we ready for them? If change is to happen in my lifetime, it needs to start now, not in five or ten years. Recently I saw the singer Anohni perform in concert. She's a trans woman, and she told stories about many of her trans friends and lovers who took their own lives. She described it as a liberation instead of a tragedy. "I would rather dash my body against the rocks than have to end my days in a repugnant heterosexual rest home," she said.

I hope that as my years continue to advance, I can face whatever comes with the same steely stare I have used to get me to this point. I worry that I won't when it comes to it. There's a small piece of toxic masculinity inside me that thinks I must still face the future – death – with stoicism and strength, when in fact the thought of it makes me want to crumple to the floor and sob. I hope I have the courage to explore this and examine what might get me closer to a place of acceptance; and if that is not possible, how I could go down in a blaze of glory instead of a puddle of tears.

I score my mortality as a 5. Death terrifies me. Well, my own does. Sometimes I just can't believe that the world will go on without me. I really want to do more work on this because time is ticking and I want to see each passing year as a blessing, not a signal of impending doom.

What do you score your mortality?

....

Why that number?

....

....

....

....

....

What would you like to work on?

....

....

....

....

....

....

YOUR QUEER WHEEL OF MIDLIFE

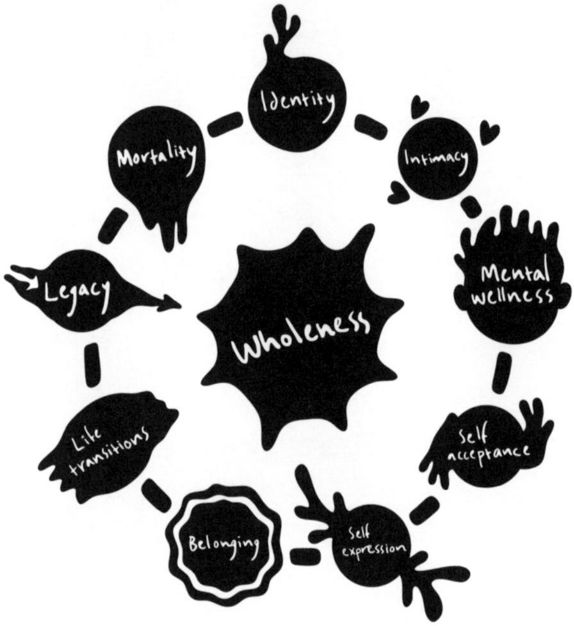

	Notes	Score
Identity		
Intimacy		
Mental Wellbeing		

Self-Acceptance		
Self-Expression		
Belonging		
Life Transitions		
Legacy		
Mortality		

REFLECTING ON THE QUEER WHEEL OF MIDLIFE

Now that you have explored the nine facets of The Queer Wheel of Midlife, you might be a little clearer about some of the areas you'd like to be more in touch with. The space below is for you to write about it. Consider the following questions:

- What do you want to dive more deeply into?
- What surprised you about your wheel?
- Where are you able to validate the strengths you already have?
- What might help you take the next bold step toward wholeness?

Now it's time to move into Part II: STILL QUEER! This includes The Queer Wholeness Method, a set of experiences and experiments to connect you with your deep and unshakeable wholeness, which will give you the power to move you toward where you want to be.

PART II

STILL QUEER!

“I like couples’ therapy. It was our wedding gift to ourselves.”

– SOPHIE, 43

THE QUEER WHOLENESS METHOD

> “I'm very mindful about protecting my peace in a way that I think I used to take for granted when I was younger. My Blackness is vilified. My femininity is vilified double-time. I'm a working parent. I'm queer. I am actively practising giving myself grace."
>
> – CHLOË, 42

Well done on making it this far, both in terms of the book and life in general! The Queer Wheel of Midlife helped us locate where we are. The next step of the process helps to locate how we are in relation to our own sense of wholeness. Middle age can present us with unique and unexpected opportunities and challenges in how we wish to live our lives today and into our own elderhood. It's a chance to reflect on what happened to get us here. Is where we are where we want to be? Midlife is the time when we can ask ourselves, *What can I do that will help me live more deliberately in the next phase of my life? How can I create the future I desire and deserve?*

Of course, everyone's experiences are unique to them. We all grow up in different places with different people around us. Our lives are influenced by a wide range of external factors outside our control: class, education, money, politics, expectations and culture, to name just a few. Our internal senses of self are also affected by how others perceive us, whether that's because of the colour of our skin, our ability to navigate through the world, the shapes of our bodies, how we think about things and who we love.

Because we are individually unique, there could be a temptation to say, "Sort yourself out," as nobody else can. But on the other hand, we could believe that, actually, we're not special at all. Everyone is influenced by everything to varying extents; therefore, everything we go through has been experienced by someone else at some time in the past or will be in the future.

Midlife queers are human snow ploughs, as we have cleared the way for the next generation of queer people. I could not be happier for the kids growing up now who celebrate Pride month at school or show up to the Prom in matching dresses with their date. You're welcome. We hopefully cleared some of the debris from the path to make it slightly less treacherous for you to walk in those heels. Of course, we aren't the first generation of snow ploughs. Queer people before us gave their lives so that we could live without fear of jail or being fired or beaten to death, to live openly as ourselves, to marry, to serve in the armed forces, to donate blood, to have children, to be elected to government, to host a talk show or to compete in the Olympics ... the idea of being able to do any of those things when I was a child was unimaginable. Of course, things are still not as okay as they should be. Far from it. Queer people, especially those who are trans, are still being murdered, regardless of their age. While it may be the case that things are getting better in general, there are pockets of our community where things are worse than ever.

The snow ploughs pushed harder and faster to clear the obstacles. It still makes my head spin. I am living a life today that I never believed would be possible or available to me. Of course, around the world, there are still many places where the life I have the privilege of living is not readily – legally or socially – available, so we must never take for granted the rights given to us that could so quickly and easily be taken away. I know how fortunate I am to have been born in a particular place at a particular time, neither of which had anything to do with me.

So, how might I make the most of my circumstances? How might more wholeness feel? I would love to be able to more easily access the innate sense of rightness that I was born with. I know that work is needed for that to be possible.

NAVIGATING THE QUEER WHOLENESS METHOD

> "I feel like I'm in the best place I've ever been in many respects, which is nice. A lot of people don't get to experience or feel that. I work hard. I'm married. We have a nice time. It's lovely."
>
> – PAUL, 53

The Queer Wholeness Method is a guided process for becoming, feeling and being whole. It contains both tasks to complete and processes to think about and observe; following it allows an unfolding of new knowledge about yourself, as well as a confirmation and validation of the qualities and strengths you may have known about but forgotten over time. How can we best get ready for it?

There are three main steps in The Queer Wholeness Method, which are broken down into smaller tasks. Each of the tasks within the three steps is an opportunity for you to find a deeper connection to your wholeness. Some of the experiences are small and fast. Others may take more time and ask for a slower quality of attention. They all add something to the process of rediscovering our wholeness. You can work through the method at your own pace. There is no rush.

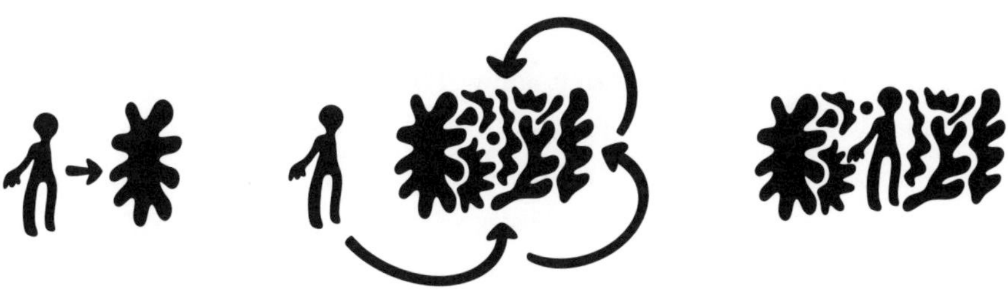

Step 1: Becoming

The first step of The Queer Wholeness Method – **Becoming** – is our starting place. The sections of Becoming are:

- **Locating your whole**: how to connect with your wholeness
- **Exploring your whole**: how to discover the different parts of wholeness
- **Understanding your whole**: how to make sense of what wholeness reveals

You will emerge from the first step with a clearer understanding of what helps and hinders your connection to wholeness. You will have explored new ways to connect with yourself at a deeper and more nuanced level, examining how your relationship to wholeness has been shaped, how to navigate barriers that may emerge in the future.

Step 2: Feeling

The second step – **Feeling** – begins with a celebration of what was revealed in the Becoming step. With a clearer vision of your wholeness, you will work through three tasks aimed at enabling you to be more present and comfortable with yourself and your wholeness.

The sections of Feeling are:

- **Examining your whole**: how to treat your wholeness gently
- **Widening your whole**: how to expand and stretch the edges of your wholeness
- **Deepening your whole**: how to get to the magical core of wholeness

At the end of the Feeling step, you will have a deeper connection to your wholeness and a calmer, less critical view of how it feels to be whole. You might begin to recognize how and when you are stepping out of your wholeness and find new techniques for rediscovering it. You might even feel more expansive and open to the magic of the world.

Step 3: Being

The third and final step – **Being** – begins to examine your relationship to wholeness in the wider world. Building on and celebrating the progress made in the Feeling step, you'll go further into your identity and sense of belonging in a range of different settings. That way, you can take the magic of your wholeness into relationships and communities beyond yourself.

The sections of Being are:

- **Expressing your whole**: how to live your queer wholeness out loud
- **Owning your whole**: how to overcome the shame of wholeness
- **Sharing your whole**: how to deepen your wholeness through connection to others

At the end of the Being step, you will have a greater sense of how you might be able to live more regularly from a place of wholeness. The techniques in this step will build your confidence to talk and act from a more stable sense of self, without feeling embarrassment or falling back on self-deprecation. You will have explored how to navigate relationships that may be helping, or even hindering, your wholeness.

The Queer Wholeness Method is an experiment, a guide and a compass. It's like a cool best friend in your pocket; something you can pick up in moments of deep dark thoughts, and also when the sky is blue and full of sun. Navigating big life changes is sometimes easier when we see them as a number of smaller decisions, and The Queer Wholeness Method will help you feel more confident in those.

Using techniques based on thinking, imagining, embodying and experiencing, you'll be guided through a collection of methods: some that may feel new, while others may seem familiar to you in some ways. One of the great opportunities that arises from doing this work on your own is that you get to examine your responses to the process without having to explain, describe or justify them to anyone. Whatever happens is the right thing to happen. Nobody else needs to understand it. Part of the process is to simply notice what's going on for you, moment to moment. To get you warmed up, before you read any further, notice how you are right now. You don't need to change anything, just notice. Are you sitting, standing or lying down? What's the air around you like? Are you hungry? Where are your feet right now? How is your breath?

You'll come across plenty of these kind of prompts throughout this section. Notice how you respond to them. Do they feel inviting? Annoying? Distracting? Deepening? It's all about coming home to your whole self, the person you were before they told you to be someone else. The prompts encourage you to stop, take stock and do something. It's not just for a bit of a laugh – although I hope you find some of them fun, but to encourage a spirit of self-reflection as you journey through The Queer Wholeness Method. How far or deep you go is up to you. You might feel inspired to talk or write about it, but as I've noted already, you don't have to share anything with anyone. It's totally up to you.

GETTING YOURSELF READY

So how are you doing right now? There's no need to change a thing. Just notice.

- How does your body feel at the moment?
- What state of mind are you in?
- How are you experiencing the world today?

All of these will influence how you enter The Queer Wholeness Method.

With your answers to the above questions in mind, I wonder what conditions would suit you best when trying The Queer Wholeness Method. Take a look at the word cloud on the next page to see what might help you get the most from the practice. Circle the ones that speak to you. Add your own if you can't see them.

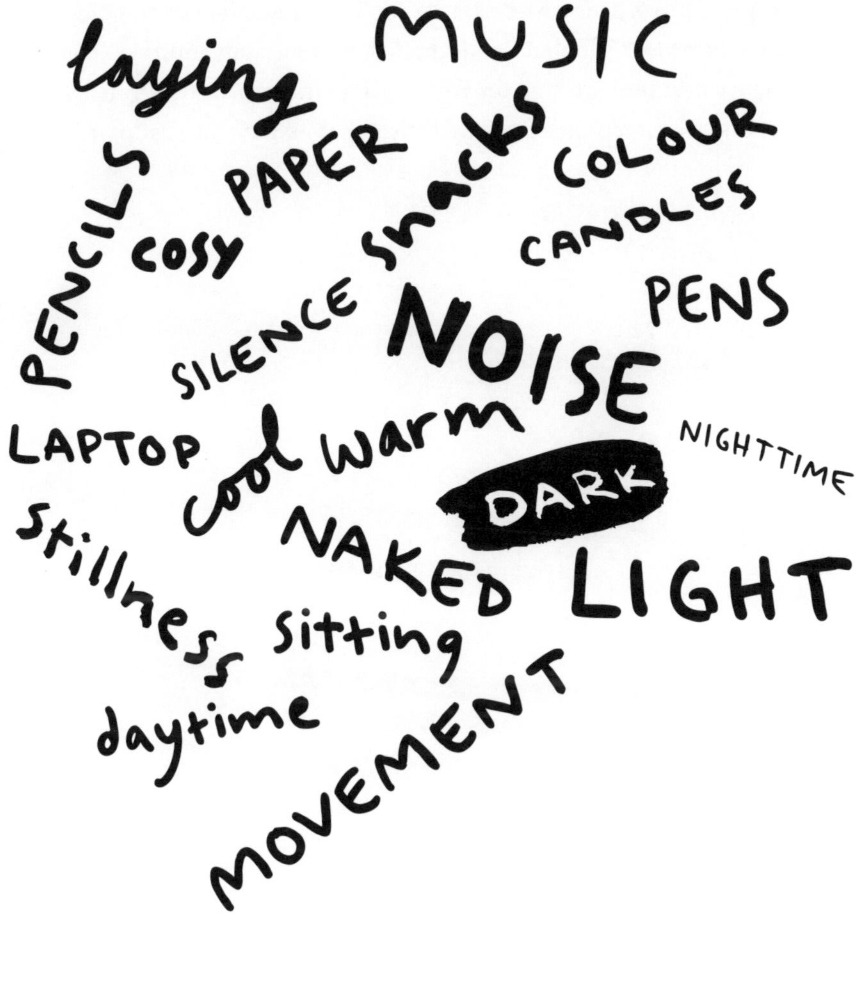
laying
MUSIC
PENCILS
PAPER
snacks
COLOUR
CANDLES
cosy
SILENCE
NOISE
PENS
LAPTOP
cool
warm
NIGHTTIME
DARK
stillness
NAKED
LIGHT
sitting
daytime
MOVEMENT

Before you start The Queer Wholeness Method I'd like to invite you to be deliberate about what feels good, or doesn't, and make any adjustments that may help. When you have a better understanding of the conditions that make you feel better, it's good data that you can take into the world when you put this book away.

As you enter The Queer Wholeness Method, you might be wondering what will happen when we get in there. I say "we" deliberately because I'm with you every step of the way. Nevertheless, stepping into The Queer Wholeness Method is your own adventure. What you discover in there is all for you. I believe in gradual steps, getting used to the experience little by little. That's what this first part is about.

STEP 1: BECOMING WHOLE

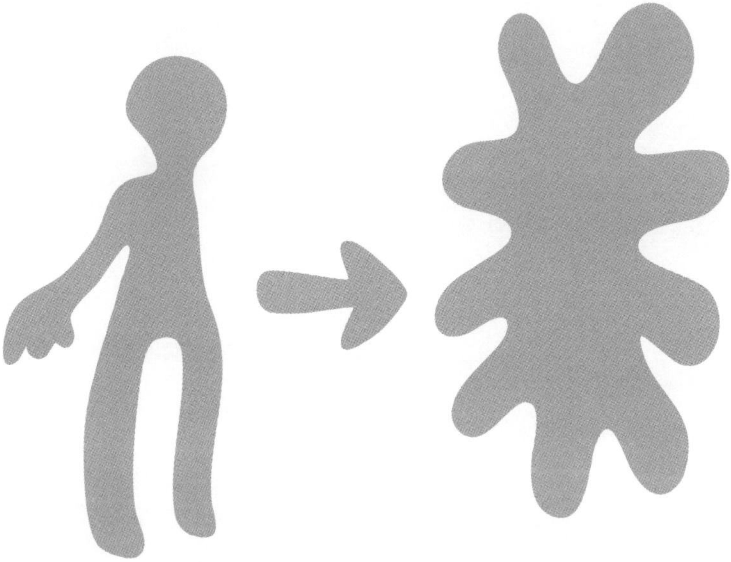

> The scaffolding is being taken away, so I feel a bit like I'm floundering at the moment. There's just too much to cope with. And I'm definitely not having enough sex."
>
> – JUSTIN, 48

Begin by asking yourself: what would you like to discover if you became more connected to your wholeness?

. . . .

. . . .

. . . .

. . . .

. . . .

. . . .

. . . .

. . . .

. . . .

. . . .

. . . .

. . . .

. . . .

. . . .

. . . .

LOCATING

Locating your whole: how to connect to your wholeness

“Remember The Incredible Hulk? I remember watching that as a very small child. And when he changed into the green Hulk, there was just something about him that was mesmerizing, and I

> wouldn't have thought in terms of sex. But I remember kissing my wall, pretending it was him."
>
> – MAXIMILIAN, 47

I spent a lot of my early years trying to find myself and understand who I am. When I managed to locate that essential aspect of me, in this case my queerness, I held it tightly. My queerness is a central pillar in who I am. I use my queerness as a north star when I feel lost. My wholeness, on the other hand, comes and goes. There's more of a dynamic distance between me and it. It's less solid and more unpredictable. At times I can sense the closeness of it, and others it feels like it exists in a different galaxy. I lose contact with it. So, how do you find something? You look for it.

That's why the first step of The Queer Wholeness Method is to find your whole. Locate it. Know where it is, so that you might speak with it, explore it and understand it better.

Your perfect wholeness

The idea of wholeness, or becoming whole, might already be so out of your experience that you may already believe that it doesn't apply to you. I'd like to try an experiment with you. Let's imagine that you have a sense of wholeness. Imagine you have had, since you were born, a completeness in who you are. A bone-deep, in-your-veins understanding that you are perfection. What's your reaction to that idea? You don't have to change or judge whatever comes up, just be aware of it. However you respond, it's good data. It means there's information there to do something with.

Drawing yourself

Before we can find your whole, you need to locate yourself. Here, I'd like you to draw a picture of yourself as you are right now. Nobody will see it except for you, so it doesn't need to be a good piece of art by anyone's standards (even your own). You can use any materials you like. There is no way to get this wrong.

When I look at my drawing, it's probably quite a good representation of how I think I look, in that perfect human shape, when in reality I look quite different. My limbs are not long, and my body is not slim. I added my tattoos, as they're part of my skin, and then I drew a pair of shorts. I added some cool trainers, a beard, a smile and my eyes and ears.

As you look at your drawing, ask yourself the following questions:

- What did you include and what did you leave out?

- Would people recognize it as you? (Keep in mind that how we see ourselves can be quite different to how others see us, which in turn can be different to how we actually are.)
- What do you feel when you look at this representation of yourself that you created?
- Does your drawing of yourself hold an emotional quality?
- What is it transmitting into the world?

Now you've started the process and have found yourself looking at an image of yourself on a page. Where could that take you? In the next step, we'll move into an exploration of your wholeness.

EXPLORING

Exploring your whole

> "I grew up in the generation where queer was an insult. I could have had way more fun if I'd been a bit more confident when I was younger. Now there's a realization that although we have a finite amount of time, there are so many more possibilities to explore."
>
> – JON, 47

How does your whole relate to your self?

I'd like you to look around you and find an object, something that might represent an idea of wholeness. You might choose something because of its shape or its colour. Maybe it has a texture you love or a comforting smell. Find something that, to you, says "whole". If you don't see one, maybe venture out and look for an item that catches your eye.

Now, let's place the object that represents your wholeness somewhere in relation to the drawing you made of yourself in the last step. Put it somewhere that shows your relationship to your wholeness. Sketch the scene in the box below.

In my drawing, my self and my whole are both on the same table, at the same level. There's approximately 18 inches between them. My self can see my whole, clearly. There's nothing in the space to obscure its view. It's static though, so my self can only see the part of my whole that's facing it. There's a huge hemisphere of whole that it can't see.

To be where I would like it to be, my self needs to invite my whole to get closer. My self needs to move around it, explore it. My whole wants to be understood, but it can't be properly known until it is examined further. My self knows where my whole is. There's a connection. I would like it to be even better.

Now, look back at your drawing – what do you think it means? Ask yourself the following questions:

- What does this experiment reveal about your self's relationship with your whole?
- How would you want it to be?
- What might have to happen to get an even deeper connection between yourself and your whole?

If you need to explore this in a different way, examine the item you found to represent wholeness. Really get into it and describe every detail you can about it. Then, compare all the little details to your own wholeness.

In my case, I found a small globe of the Earth, which immediately made me think of wholeness.

Like the globe, my whole contains a lot of detail. Some of it is in a language I don't understand, but I get the general meaning of what it represents. There is no right way up to my whole. It should, and could, be seen from any angle. My whole represents a lot of places, territories, terrains and borders. My whole has different temperatures and weather conditions. It can provide the conditions for life to thrive. My whole shows me where I have been, but not yet where I am going. It helps me understand where I am. Unlike the globe, I don't believe my whole is hollow, but it's also not solid inside. It has space for everything to move around together. My whole also feels smaller than this globe, like I could hold it tightly in two hands.

And you? What have you discovered as you explored your whole?

UNDERSTANDING

Understanding your whole

> "It took me another couple of years to come out and tell everybody else. I had been doing it in secret, gay by night, straight by day, kind of like a Batman of shame."
>
> – CRAIG, 51

Understanding something is an active process. To understand an issue or a thing, we have to be with it, experience it, think about it and ask questions of it. The process of understanding comes from a place of data collection and analysis, creating new knowledge about it, making meaning from it and then taking some utility from it that can be applied in a future scenario. Understanding means connecting the dots.

So far, you have located your whole and maybe got a sense of where you are with it. You might have a better feel for the distance you are from it and what it needs from you to be even more embedded and embodied. You've explored it, contemplated its qualities and maybe even begun to see some similarities and differences that make you curious.

Our approach to understanding our wholes begins by knowing what we know. For me, for example, I now know that:

- I have a good view of my whole, but I can't see it all.
- I know what it is and where it is, and I'd like to know it better.
- It is light, with lots of detail on the surface and interesting stuff inside.
- It contains information on where I have been and where I am now.
- It can be held any way up.

To create some new knowledge from my whole, I can now ask questions of it. The questions I would like to pose to my whole are:

- How might I get to know you better?
- What are the risks and benefits to opening you up?
- Looking at my path so far, where do you think I might go next?
- When will I be ready to look at the hidden parts?

Using these questions, I imagined the following conversation with my whole:

Me: How might I know you better?
My whole: You need to hold me more often now that I'm here. You can talk to me, and I will respond. You know where I am now. You want to know what I look like or how I feel? Just talk to me.

Me: What are the risks and benefits to opening you up?
My whole: One of the risks is that I fall apart, that I get destroyed, that I stopped being useful. The benefit of opening me up is that you get to see inside. There's also an understanding and then intelligence of knowing you already know what's inside.

Me: Looking at my path so far, where do you think I might go next?
My whole: Your path so far is a map of where you've been. But that excludes a lot. It doesn't tell you why. You made the decisions to go where you went. I know that those decisions were right for you at the time. They were the only decisions that you could make in terms of where you went next. Now, the opportunity is to make some different decisions, ones that get you to where you want to go. The question is, do you know where you want to go?

Me: When will I be ready to look at the hidden parts?
My whole: You are already ready; and you will never be ready.

Readiness is not the issue. Hidden parts hold power, meaning, significance, fear, shadows – things you don't want people to see, maybe including yourself. Know that by showing yourself those hidden parts, you understand yourself better, and that you may show others so they may feel able to look at their own.

Now, it's your turn. Record a conversation between you and your whole, asking it these questions:

- How might I get to know you better?
- What are the risks and benefits to opening you up?
- Looking at my path so far, where do you think I might go next?
- When will I be ready to look at the hidden parts?

How does your whole answer?

. . . .

. . . .

. . . .

. . . .

. . . .

What can you take from the conversation with your whole?

. . . .

. . . .

. . . .

. . . .

. . . .

. . . .

What do you understand now?

. . . .

. . . .

. . . .

. . . .

. . . .

. . . .

Now that you have located, explored and understood your whole, ask yourself ...

- How does your wholeness support your queerness?
- Has anything unexpected emerged from the process so far?
- What are you learning about your wholeness and your queerness?

STEP 2: FEELING WHOLE

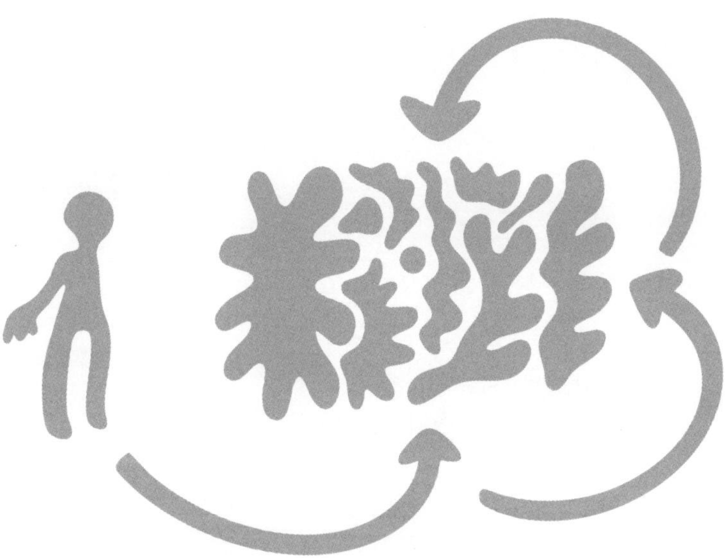

> My dad was talking to me on a flight back from Greece about seven years ago. He said to me, 'Have you had a good holiday?', and I said, 'Yeah, it just would have been nice to share it with someone.' At which point he said, 'Have you ever thought about being with a woman?'"

– CHARLIE, 45

How would you like to feel if you were more deeply connected to your wholeness?

. . . .

. . . .

. . . .

. . . .

. . . .

. . . .

. . . .

. . . .

. . . .

. . . .

. . . .

ENJOYING

Enjoying your whole

> "I love being queer because of our contribution to the world. We've given so much in terms of the arts and literature. We're moving it forward, where straight people would just be left behind in the dark."
>
> – SALIM, 45

It has taken half a century for me to begin the process of feeling whole. The 1970s and '80s were not exactly known for tolerance of queerness and I was fortunate to be a teenager at a time when the beginnings of a shift in society were taking place. As I entered adulthood, many of the legal and cultural barriers to queer wholeness began to fall away but there was still a backdrop of hostility. The last quarter of a century has seen seismic shifts forward in equality, and as queer people we are more visible, present and influential. Despite this, more and more of us queer folk who are well into our adulthood are struggling with who we are.

As a coach and mentor, I see queer people who, on the surface, are living their best lives: artists, performers, CEOs, parents. Underneath the surface, not very far down, lurk doubt, shame, fear, guilt, hopelessness and low self-esteem. Often, when I'm working with someone, I can see that deep down they know they are really and truly whole, but they just don't feel it. They can't access the bright glowing fire of wholeness that exists inside them.

Enjoying our whole is one way of feeling it better. To enjoy something means looking at or considering it carefully, thoughtfully and in detail and taking in all the delicious goodness that it offers. Enjoying something is a way to get to know better the function and purpose of a thing and how it brings us joy. Through enjoying our whole, we can more closely and clearly explain it, know it and have options for what to do with it.

Your wholeness festival

Imagine your wholeness decided to throw itself a festival. It can be as big as Glastonbury, or something you hold in your own back garden.

- What would the stages be called?
- What bands represent the best of your wholeness? (These can be real artists or imagined ones!)
- What is the vibe of the wholeness festival?
- How might you create the most wonderful experience to enjoy your wholeness?

What does your festival map look like? Draw it in the box.

This is how I imagine my wholeness festival:

1. The resilience stage

This stage is dedicated to those who have faced significant adversity and come out stronger. It's about celebrating the power of survival, endurance, and the ability to thrive despite challenges.

- **The Warriors' Choir** A group performance symbolizing the collective strength of those who have lived through the AIDS crisis, discrimination and personal trauma, coming together to sing anthems of hope and perseverance
- **Phoenix Rising** A solo artist who has rebuilt their life after hitting rock bottom, sharing songs of rebirth and new beginnings
- **The Reflectors** An introspective folk duo that plays acoustic sets, exploring themes of self-reflection, recovery and healing

2. The expression stage

This stage showcases artists who have embraced their identities fully and use self-expression as a form of empowerment. It's colourful, bold and unapologetic.

- **Tattooed Truths** A punk band with members who each use their bodies as canvases, expressing their identities through tattoos, piercings and personal stories
- **The Nonconformists** A gender-fluid collective that blends genres like pop, rock and electronic music, celebrating the freedom to be who you are without limits
- **The Late Bloomers** An ensemble of performers who came out later in life, now revelling in the joy of self-discovery and expressing themselves through vibrant, eclectic fashion and music

3. The community stage

This stage focuses on the themes of community, belonging and the complexities of fitting in or standing out. It's a mix of joyous celebration and thoughtful exploration of what it means to belong.

- **Chosen Family** A collective that sings about the importance of creating your own community and the bonds that go beyond blood ties
- **The Outsiders** An alternative rock band that plays songs about the struggles of fitting in, both in queer spaces and the wider world, with anthems for those who have always felt on the fringes
- **The Safe Spaces** A chill, ambient group that creates a soundscape meant to evoke feelings of security, acceptance and home within the LGBTQ+ community

4. The legacy stage

This stage is dedicated to those who are contemplating their legacy and the meaning of life as they grow older. It's a reflective and poignant space, with performances that honour the past and look to the future.

- **The Storytellers** A folk group composed of older LGBTQ+ individuals who share life stories through song, touching on themes of mortality, memory and legacy
- **The Keepers of Time** A band that blends traditional and modern music to explore the passage of time, with lyrics that reflect on what we leave behind and how we are remembered
- **The Future Ancestor** A solo artist who sings about the duality of living in the present, while being mindful of the impact they wish to leave on the next generation

I picture myself spending a long weekend at this festival. The people attending are smiling, feeling joy and sharing love. There are plenty of places to sit down, as it's tiring to stand up all day! The food is good, and the sun is shining. I feel like I can be myself here.

Now, think back to the festival you've devised.

- What does the lineup of your festival inspire in you?
- How would you like to show up to your festival?
- In what ways could you enjoy yourself more fully?

DEEPENING

Deepening your whole

> "I never used to think about dying, but even my mother was like, 'You're going to die of AIDS,' just because I was gay. I'm positive now, I have been for nine years, and maybe it triggered me to turn myself round a bit. Do something with more meaning."
>
> – SAM, 43

Going deeper into something helps us grow. One of the ways to deepen our whole is to consider it through the lens of art. Images and artworks can help us make meaning, to get closer to the soul of our whole. When I say "art", it doesn't have to involve an expensive trip to the Louvre and three nights in a four-star hotel, although if that's what you have in mind, you do you.

Visual inspiration

Spend a few minutes noticing the images around you right now. Maybe there's a print on the wall, or the cover of a book on a shelf. If something catches your eye, it wants you to see it.

For this experiment, you can use anything with an image on it: some old birthday cards, postcards you've collected, fridge magnets, posters hanging in town or even a Google image search. Make a sketch of it here.

Stand as close to your inspiration image – or hold it as close to yourself – as possible, so you can really inspect all of the details. Now, step back and notice if you can see the entire image at once without focusing on a particular part of it. Finally, consider these questions – and write your answers in the box below.

- What properties does the image have?
- Do you notice shapes or textures?
- Does it bring up any emotions for you?

Now, imagine the image is the answer to the following question: how do I increase the depth, intensity or complexity of my whole? Give yourself time to see how the image answers the question. Make some notes below.

When I tried this experiment, I found a sticker on my notebook, a small UFO beaming a rainbow onto the earth. I jotted down the qualities of my rainbow UFO, which were:

- Simple lines
- Clear shapes
- Bold colours
- Bright and vivid
- Representation of something alien
- Positive vibes
- Shiny
- Windows to see out of and into
- A bridge / control deck
- A white outline

My rainbow UFO gives me the permission to:

- Believe that there is intelligent life out there
- Come in peace
- Boldly go where no-one has gone before
- Live long and prosper

The rainbow UFO tells me I can increase the depth, intensity or complexity of my whole by:

- Being bold in my alienness
- Showing my rainbow colours vividly
- Shining a positive light
- Holding many possibilities

If those are the answers to how I increase the depth of my wholeness, I wonder how I might embody them and integrate them into my daily life? The invitations to be bold and vivid bring up some vulnerability around visibility. If aliens did land on Earth, would we welcome them with open arms or immediately become aggressive to them? Maybe I'm not brave enough right now to live from this place of wholeness. After all, it's an ongoing process, not a quick fix.

Before we close this experiment, look back at your image and ask yourself one last question: what might it reveal for you in its wisdom?

STROKING

Stroking your whole

> When is the guilt going to go? When will the shame disappear? Me and my husband have been together for 18 years, but we never

> hold hands in public. It's not because we don't want to, we're just so programmed to not reveal anything."
>
> – MIKE V, 52

Dan and I were staying in a hotel for a friend's 50th birthday last year. It was, granted, in a very conservative town, and we left it late to book somewhere to stay, so we had to make do with the local pub-chain hotel. We were waiting to check in behind a straight couple who were enjoying some light-hearted banter with the receptionist who was a young lad, apparently comfortable to have a laugh with the customers. He waved them off and then it was our turn. I noticed he was wearing a bodycam around his neck, which was, in hindsight, a red flag. When I gave my name for the reservation, he looked at us both, puzzled, and said, "Just the one room?" I replied, "Yes, that's what we had booked." "Do you need two beds?" he asked. "No, we're married," I replied. He looked flustered but said, "Oh, that's okay, you just didn't mention it on the booking form." Maybe I completed it in a hurry, but I don't remember seeing the gay / straight tick box. Dan and I were giving each other telepathic signals and doing the eye-rolling thing that is so familiar to all of us queer folk. I quickly made the decision to get this over with as soon as possible. I said nothing else, collected our key and we walked to our room. There was a distinct lack of banter.

Lying on the bed, I felt confused, angry and disempowered. What stopped me from pointing out the difference in the way he checked us in compared to the straight couple before us? He didn't ask them if they needed two beds, or point out that they had only booked one room. Maybe they were brother and sister, but he didn't ask if they had ticked that box. I decided I would email the company to complain, not in an annoying way, but as a helpful, "here's how it could be better next time" tone. I wondered how the receptionist would respond if his manager called him in for a chat and said, "We've had a complaint." Would they collude and laugh it off, or would he see the impact of his behaviour and actually learn a different way of being around queer folk? Would he send us an apology? I never found out – as time passed and it felt like I was making a big deal out of it, I didn't bother sending the email. The fact that I let it go makes me feel even worse now. Not only did I ignore an opportunity to say something at the time, I also failed to follow up.

When I told people about the experience, they were outraged, agreeing how terrible it was. None of us could believe it happened in this day and age. The thing is, I didn't just believe it, I was waiting for it to happen. I think it is going to happen every single time we check into a hotel together, and it surprises me when it doesn't. I have absorbed so much negativity toward queer people in my life that my default position is to assume people are homophobic and then be pleasantly surprised if they're not. It can be exhausting to face these situations, however regularly or irregularly they happen. It has happened all my life.

How does this fit with the idea of Queer Wholeness? Isn't this a bit of a downer after discovering so much positivity?

I believe that part of my wholeness is the ability not just to forgive people who act badly toward me, but to also forgive myself for the times I accepted it. For all the moments when I could have said something but chose not to. The situations when I was just too tired to do the right thing. Queer Wholeness is the ability to be compassionate to ourselves. To stroke our whole when it feels tender or bruised.

SHOWING COMPASSION TO YOURSELF

Make a list of some of the times you remember when someone said or did something to you that you felt was homophobic / transphobic / generally queer-negative.

Next to that, write down what you said or did in the moment.

In the third column, write down what you wish you had said.

What happened?	What did I do or say?	What do I wish I had done or said?

Next to each entry, give yourself a love heart, or a kiss, or a smiley face. Send love to the self who was just too tired to say something that day. Be compassionate to the person who knew what they wanted to say, but at that moment just didn't feel safe enough. Stroke the soft underbelly of the self who learned, through no fault of its own, that sometimes keeping quiet is the only option. There is little point expecting others to be kind to us if we can't be kind to ourselves. We may not have had this modelled for us or been taught that it is the right thing to do, but it's never too late to understand, forgive and soothe ourselves for making the choices we felt were the only ones available to us in a particular moment. Maybe we could soften the tone of our own critical voices, even a little.

Imagine how it would be if we achieved this even just some of the time. It doesn't mean we have to always get it right. In fact, I would hate to have to see myself as any kind of good example of anything. Instead, I would find it freeing to believe that I could meet my shortcomings with a gentle acceptance. If my default mode switched from self-judging and regretting to taking a measured and informed view of my capacity to respond in the moment, offering kindness where needed, I would see that as a superpower of queer wholeness.

Becoming and feeling more whole

Before we move to the final step of The Queer Wholeness Method, take a moment to note what you are discovering about yourself so far.

What are you sitting with as you have been becoming and feeling more whole?

STEP 3: BEING WHOLE

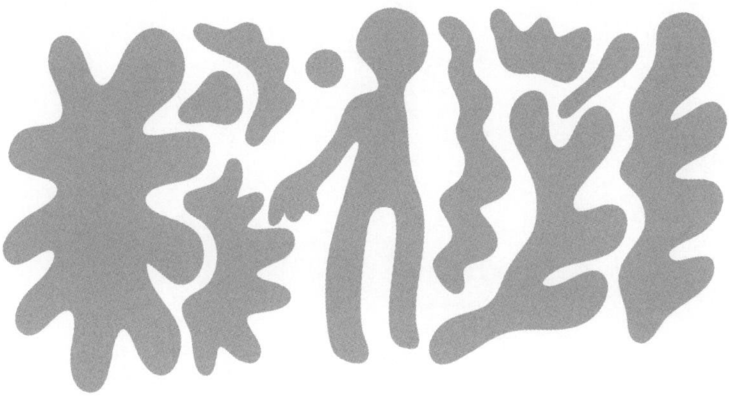

"I enjoy having sex with much older men, because they tend to be a lot better at it. Well, they tend to be more attentive than younger men, who feel like sometimes they're trying to drill a new hole."

– WILLIAM, 40

What possibilities might you encounter if you experienced what it means to truly be whole?

. . . .

. . . .

. . . .

. . . .

. . . .

. . . .

. . . .

. . . .

. . . .

EXPRESSING

Expressing your whole

> "I'm genuinely proud of my evolution and who I've become. I feel really content. I am an open person and I wear my heart on my sleeve. It helps being naked on the beach because I'm 100 per cent authentic. That was a revelation to me."
>
> – DAVE, 46

In our first year of secondary school, they decided to take individual as well as class photos. To this day I'm not great with being photographed, as I have no facial range and my standard response when a camera is pointed at me is to smile like a muppet. Being photogenic is not one of my natural gifts. When I look at that individual school photo, I come across as so awkward. My hands are half-clasped in my lap. I remember my trousers being self-consciously too tight. My hair screams neither boy nor girl. I am smiling but inside I'm terrified of being really seen. As the years have passed, I've become better at expressing myself, but it still takes work. There's a part of me that's still a chubby 11-year-old, squinting into the lens, wishing it was over.

When we start really seeing and believing our own worth, we cultivate stronger senses of self-esteem and confidence. We feel empowered as we confidently navigate and overcome everyday barriers and challenges. This helps us foster hope and growth within and finally find the strength to effectively help, be with, serve and lead others. I believe we do this by reconnecting with our wholeness. We become, feel and take nourishment from being whole. By accepting, embracing and celebrating our wholeness, we can add a little more love into the world and that includes self-love. When it's difficult to accept ourselves, we might deny aspects of our identity or personality and that makes it easier for us to fit in or be accepted by others. Doing this fractures our wholeness.

When we are fractured, we feel incomplete, inauthentic, unhappy or dissatisfied. We can't focus. We don't think creatively. We give ourselves a hard time for every little thing that goes wrong. I have, at various points in my life, accepted and rejected so many different bits of myself. Maybe for a while I hated my body, and then I didn't. For a period of time, I was confident and sociable, and then I wasn't. Wholeness for me has never been static. To be whole is to embrace the ebb and flow of life, the inhale and exhale of living. Sometimes the tides threaten to drown us. Other times we float calmly on the surface of a warm pool. Throughout it all, our wholeness never changes. We are always whole – we just don't always feel it. Instead, we are in a process of being, feeling and staying whole against the backdrop of a world that does not respect or revere us.

Expanding your expression

This next experiment is one of both generating a lot of data in a fixed amount of time, and appreciating that even the smallest amount of time is long enough to work on our whole. Expressing something is the way we convey thoughts, ideas and feelings to others. Sometimes finding the language to do this can limit us, or we overthink it trying to get the perfect answer. As an experiment in expressing our whole, we're going to use a technique from improvization that I've adapted. If you were to use it in a more traditional way, you might ask how many uses can I find for a pen in one minute. Nothing is off limits. Yes, I can write with it, and I can conduct an orchestra with it, or use it as a replacement chopstick or prodder for slow walkers. You get the idea.

Find a timer (sand, clock or phone), and set yourself an amount of time that adds a little pressure. Maybe no more than three minutes. When you start the timer, in three minutes you need to come up with as many ways to finish one of the following sentences:

- My queer whole is ...
- My queer whole is like ...

You can take inspiration from the space you're in, the things around you or whatever comes to your mind. There are no wrong answers. Make a note of what happens.

....

....

....

....

....

....

....

....

....

I used a timer, which turned out to be four minutes. I tried hard not to censor myself, so I recorded myself walking around my space, describing my queer whole in the style of anything that caught my eye, or made me think of an idea.

- My queer whole is like a Trojan horse – it contains multitudes.
- My queer whole is expressed in primary colours.
- My queer whole is like fireworks going off at night.
- My queer whole synthesizes light.
- My queer whole sometimes makes me tired.
- My queer whole is like an advancing storm with waves crashing onto land.
- My queer whole is like the comforting purr of a cat.
- My queer whole is the face of a wolf protecting its pack.
- My queer whole enjoys connection.
- My queer whole is ancient.
- My queer whole is magical.
- My queer whole is art.
- My queer whole has vulnerability.
- My queer whole is solid.
- My queer whole is like scales, weighing truth and fairness.
- My queer whole has a secret compartment.
- My queer whole contains volumes.
- My queer whole is terrifying.
- My queer whole is like an archway.
- My queer whole is like a cracked piece of stone.
- My queer whole is allergic to boring.
- My queer whole is like a map of the world.
- My queer whole shelters me.
- My queer whole is learning a different language.
- My queer whole is a collection of work.
- My queer whole is a place where people can gather.
- My queer whole is a caricature of something else.
- My queer whole is light.

- My queer whole is sometimes kept in the corner behind the door.
- My queer whole is recognizable.
- My queer whole is like a throne upon which the queen can sit.
- My queer whole is quality.
- My queer whole is curated.
- My queer whole is precious.
- My queer whole is cool.
- My queer whole is like royalty.
- My queer whole is breakable.
- My queer whole is like caramel.
- My queer whole is a fairy tale.
- My queer whole is like gold gilded on precious fabric.
- My queer whole is power.
- My queer whole is electric.

When reading through the list, several statements stood out. They made me wonder, ask questions and get curious. But let's look at these three in particular:

- My queer whole is allergic to boring.
- My queer whole is a caricature of something else.
- My queer whole has a secret compartment.

How might I express my wholeness in a way that isn't boring? What is my wholeness a caricature of? What's inside the secret compartment of my wholeness?

Once you've considered the statements that give you pause, take some of the most impactful, positive or meaningful sentences and re-label them as "My queerness is". In my case, some of my sentences read:

- My queerness is power.
- My queerness is light.

- My queerness is magical.
- My queerness is ancient.
- My queerness is art.

If I let those settle, I notice a feeling of rightness. I know, at a deep level, that those statements are true, yet I would have taken longer than four minutes to think of them. I may not even have dared to believe them or say them. Seeing them in writing solidifies them. They are real. This is how I express my whole.

It's an interesting experience to get the answer to a question so clearly defined. In a way, it's easier to be in a place of not knowing. When you have the solutions, you become the question.

- Will I or won't I?
  - If I do, what might go well or badly?
  - If I don't, what does that say about me?
- Do these really belong to me?
  - If not, what can I do to feel more closeness to my wholeness?
- In other words, how do I own it?

OWNING

Owning your whole

> "We grew up hiding, faking it and putting a mask on. We basically buried a massive aspect of ourselves, which is borderline psychological damage, to the point where I'm still trying to figure out where my identity sits."
>
> – NEIL, 48

How many times has someone paid you a compliment, only for you to reject it? I do it less than I used to after a friend pointed out how disrespectful it was of me to disagree with her truth. She said I was a good coach, and in response, I rambled on about how it was really just luck and working with good clients and really anyone could do it. She replied with: "Well, I'll just take my fucking compliment and go sit in the bin with it, shall I?" That sentence started to shift how I see compliments, and feedback in general. Feedback is a gift, and like all gifts, we can return them, give them to someone else, throw them away or treasure them forever.

Society rarely had positive expectations for someone who came out at the time we did. Nobody ever told me that being queer was a good thing. I was never allowed to believe that anyone would ever see me as someone they would want to be like. Maybe for other reasons, like if I was good at maths (which I was until it got complicated), or if I baked a good cake (slightly dodgy but on the right track), but never for my queerness – the thing that played, and plays, such a huge part of who I am. In middle age, I do believe that I have a better relationship with my queerness in a way that would never have felt possible to my younger self. I love my queerness. I would not change it for the world. Yet the world disagrees and would probably prefer if I kept it to myself and stopped talking about it.

Can you own your queerness?

On some level, I know and believe that it is still not okay or safe for me to totally own my queerness. Owning something is about having a relationship with it. More than that, it's about having a good relationship with it, and that takes time, energy and commitment. Communication is key. I don't often talk to myself, so to get to know my queerness better, I'm going to take my whole for a walk. They do it all the time in shows like *The West Wing* when they say, "Walk with me." All the best conversations happen on the move. Standing shoulder-to-shoulder somehow makes it easier to say the things we might not feel comfortable saying while looking into someone's eyes.

So, I'm going on a walking date with my whole as a way of understanding it better, knowing its purpose and appreciating its value.

If we have the ability, walking and talking is one of the most simple tools we have. Even if we're not able to walk, we might be able to move in different ways. Movement through space gives a different texture to our thinking. I swim most days, and it's where I come up with some of my best ideas for my writing. There is something about the combination of being supported with some resistance and moving in a forward direction that seems to generate good creativity.

Walking with your whole

In whichever way you prefer to move, I invite you to take your whole for a chat.

I did this experiment during a writing retreat in Barcelona. I felt so lucky to be there. The scenery was beautiful, and the grounds were perfect for exploring. The owners had made a labyrinth from stones on one section of the garden. I had always pictured a labyrinth to be like a maze with a hot Minotaur in the middle, but this was simply a spiral of stones with a sign that encouraged you to walk it. I decided this was where I should speak to my whole.

I walked the labyrinth twice. The first time I wanted George Michael with me, so I shuffled his songs on Spotify. On the way into the labyrinth, I got "One More Try", which is about hesitancy to start something new after being hurt. It made me walk slowly, taking my time to notice my feet and feel the ground. The song ended just as I got to the centre of the labyrinth, and as I started to make my return journey, "Outside" started playing. It's a very different vibe. It is defiant, liberated and powerful, a big "fuck you" to anyone who tries to shame us. I danced some parts of the labyrinth, smiling and laughing at the difference in my energy on the way out.

The second time I walked the labyrinth, I read my Queer Wholeness statements out loud, again and again.

My queerness is power. My queerness is light. My queerness is magical. My queerness is ancient. My queerness is art. Around and around the labyrinth, saying them again and again. A few minutes in, I said the word "ancient" and started to cry. I was connected to a deep, old kind of magic that reminded me queer people have been here since the dawn of time. Walking this circle of stones, repeating those sentences, was like casting a spell, invoking all my queer ancestors to be with me, to walk with me. When I reached the centre, I felt a little dizzy. I stood still and pressed my feet into the earth, feeling connected and stable. Then, I said:

> I am nature, in nature. Everything about me is natural.
>
> There is nothing about this moment that needs to change. Nothing about me needs to change.

It took my breath away to say those words out loud. Nothing about me needs to change. It felt as though the words belonged to someone else, but they were mine. My queerness is mine. Nothing about me needs to change. I thanked the stones at the centre and began walking back, repeating my Queer Wholeness statements out loud again, this time in reverse order.

I had reached the exit of the labyrinth, but it was the opposite side to where I had entered, which was confusing. I could see the other side, and while I thought I had been going back in the same direction, I came out at a different point. I could see where I started, reflected on the powerful sense of acceptance that I felt in the middle, and realized now I could move in a different direction.

Where did you walk your whole?

. . . .

. . . .

. . . .

. . . .

. . . .

What new insights were revealed from the process?

. . . .

. . . .

. . . .

. . . .

. . . .

. . . .

How near or far from owning your wholeness do you feel?

. . . .

. . . .

. . . .

. . . .

. . . .

. . . .

SHOWING

Showing your whole

> "I come across as quite brash and confident but a lot of it is convincing myself. I think I'm a noisy introvert. I'm actually very happy in my own company."
>
> – JAMES, 48

On the night of my 50th birthday, my husband took me to see Madonna's Celebration Tour at the O2 Arena in London. I had already told him I didn't want a party, or to be away from home, but that it would be good to do something – just the two of us – that I would remember. Madonna was on the first leg of her Four Decades Greatest Hits Tour and it was the perfect place for me to be on that big birthday. During the fourth song, "Open Your Heart", I started to cry. It wasn't a big sobbing ugly cry, there were just a couple of tears on my face, and I was also smiling. I probably looked ridiculous, a 50-year-old man, smiling and crying and singing all at the same time.

For my 13th birthday, I was allowed to throw a party. It was the first time I had enough friends to make it worthwhile. I invited five people, they all came, and we spent a couple of hours in the evening at my house watching TV and listening to music. I rented *Ghostbusters* and *Muppet Babies* from the local video store, and we had a thoroughly wholesome time. One of my friends gifted me a box of mint Matchmakers and the 12-inch single of Madonna's "Open Your Heart", which had just been released. It had what I would still argue is the best extended version of any song ever, coming in at ten minutes long. The "Open Your Heart" video had premiered a few days before, and I immediately learned the dance routine performed by a stripper Madonna, working the booths of a peep show in a Jean Paul Gaultier corset against a backdrop of Tamara De Lempicka paintings. It was high art for pop culture.

The party was, in fact, the only one I hosted, as the years from 13 onward contained things that I didn't want my friends to witness. My parents' relationship was on the verge of collapse, and my queerness was about to explode like a pubescent Jackson Pollock. And of course, around that time, there was an atmosphere of open hostility toward queer people. I could not imagine ever coming out and living safely.

On top of all that, my mum's drinking soaked our family in sorrow and shame. I'm an only child, so there was nowhere to hide. I became a sponge and a shield for the emotional spillage caused by my mum's behaviour. I was stuck between the uncensored, unfiltered agony leaking out of my mum, and the buttoned-up, tightly held stoicism of my dad. My response was to pretend to everyone, including myself, that everything was fine. I'm sure I wasn't entirely convincing all the time, but I gave it a good shot. Every movement, word, look and comment was curated and filtered to portray a person who was totally and completely okay. Ironically, nobody ever asked me if I was okay. Our wider family was fully aware of my mum's drinking, but no-one talked about it; or if they did, they kept me out of the conversation. All of this – my mum's drinking, my parents' relationship troubles, my queerness – didn't affect my exterior. I kept smiling and showed no weakness. Vulnerability was not an option. Sure, I was being bullied every day at school, but I couldn't tell my parents about that because I might have to let them know that the reason for the bullying was my queerness. Eventually, my mum left my dad and me to move into her own flat.

I learned in those teenage years to show different parts of myself to different people, always based on my own interpretation of what was safe or not. Living at home with my dad, who I felt I had little in common with, was a lonely existence. When I went to school, I navigated between the small group of friends I had, an oasis of joy and fun, and the older kids who seemed to be waiting around every corner to intimidate and scare me. I lived moment to moment, resisting the temptation to imagine that things might possibly one day be okay, because I had absolutely zero evidence that it could possibly be true.

Luckily, I tapped into something in me that knew none of this was my fault. I refused to blame myself for the bullying or the breakups, the drama or the drinking. I had a very strong sense of self and a deep knowing that I needed to survive this. Fortunately, I was not someone who ever considered taking my own life. I believed myself to be far too important. I was able to connect to a sense of inner wholeness, an understanding that my queerness was part of me, and if people bullied me about it, they were just showing their own ignorance. I knew that my parents' relationship was their own responsibility, and I could see why they were finding it so hard to be together. Even at that age, I knew it wasn't my job to fix them. I also understood that I had very little control over anything other than myself. I exerted that control very strongly, presenting this superhero self to the world when, really, I was incredibly lost, vulnerable and afraid.

That's why, standing in the O2, singing and smiling and crying to "Open Your Heart", I couldn't quite believe that I was still here, still queer and having the time of my life. Not only had I made it to 50, I was doing pretty well in life. Madonna had dancers dressed as her younger self on stage, representing her at various points in her life. I imagined 13-year-old me at my birthday party, wearing a yellow silk shirt and purple cardigan, dancing to "Open Your Heart", containing universes of emotional turmoil that seemed to find peace when singing at the top of my lungs. I thanked 13-year-old me for still being here, dancing next to me, reminding me of how far I had come. Nevertheless, in the middle of my life, I refuse to pretend that everything was, or is, okay. I can open my heart to you, showing the whole of myself, for the very first time. It's a celebration.

The knowledge I have gained through The Queer Wholeness Method has helped me to become, feel and be whole. I recognize that I am always changing. We are always changing. Taking myself through the process again in the future will reveal new, unexpected knowing. For now, I am content that this part of the work is done.

FIND THE HEART OF YOUR WHOLE

This technique helps you find the heart of your whole. It's really simple, and all you need is a piece of paper.

Contemplate the qualities of the paper you chose.

- How does it look and feel?
- What aspects of it resonate with you?
- What similarities do you have with the paper?

Now make a fold in it. Any kind of fold, anywhere. And as you do that, contemplate something about yourself that is characteristic of you, that should be celebrated. Imagine embodying the fold in the paper with that characteristic. Next, I'd like you to remember the reason you are reading this book. Really feel the reason you arrived here. See if you notice any sensations in your body as you think about that. And make another fold in the paper, any kind of fold, anywhere. As you do that, contemplate your reason for starting the book, and your reason for staying. Maybe celebrate your progress already.

And now I'd like you to centre yourself and think about where you are today. Ask yourself, "Right now, what do I most need to receive?" Then, make another fold in the paper, any kind of fold anywhere. As you do that, seal into the paper a wish for the thing you need to receive.

And lastly, I'd like you to consider the previous year, your unique, challenging, exhilarating, difficult, fun year – or however you would describe it – and ask yourself:

- What is it about my current situation that I can imagine being grateful for in a year's time?
- What quality or strength have I been building that means in another year I will be more than I was?

Then, make another fold in the paper, any kind of fold anywhere, and as you do that, seal into the paper a promise you make to yourself.

Now, hold your paper in your hand and feel all the words and thoughts and emotions you have poured into it. See if a word comes up for you, one that captures the essence of what you're feeling right now. It will be a word you can use as a reminder of who you are, who you are becoming, what you need, and what you want.

What is that word?

. . . .

This word, if you want to, is the word you can share when people ask you what The Queer Wholeness Method is about. This is the place we have reached, together.

My word, today, is acceptance. I offer that as an invitation to all of us to consider how we might accept ourselves even more fully. More boldly. With passion and love.

So how do we show this to people? Showing our wholeness is not only a way to celebrate our beautiful queerness, it is also a lighthouse in the storm to others. So, let's now look at a practical way of living our wholeness out loud.

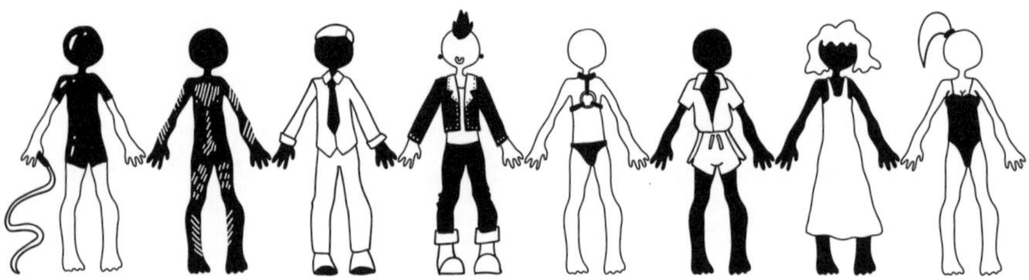

WHERE DO WE GO FROM HERE?

> “I still need a space where my sexuality is valid and not challenged. I do miss the loss of some of those spaces. People say, ‘Oh, but gay people can go anywhere now.’ Yes, we can, but you can’t have a fondle in a straight bar or a passionate kiss with someone because it’s not safe.”
>
> – MARK, 41

The next part of the book shows you how to compile your Queer Midlife Manifesto (using your results from The Queer Wholeness Method) as a way to feel a sense of achievement and accomplishment, as well as clarity over the direction you wish to live your life from here.

The aim is to bring closure to the process and allow space for insights to emerge through creating and sharing a personal manifesto – your promise to yourself.

Doing this on your own is fine, but to make it even more powerful you will be invited to be part of a global community of explorers who can help each other to become, feel and be whole.

PART III

NOW WHAT?

“I’ll give some very wise spiritual words. They go something like this: Love yourself, bitch. Love yourself. And even more importantly, like yourself. Inhabit your body. Inhabit your right to be. Inhabit your right to exist.”

– GRANT, 55

CHANGE YOUR WHOLE, CHANGE THE WORLD

> I feel like I'm having my adolescence all over again, but I feel like I'm already past it."
>
> – MIKE F, 47

So, we have all this new information about ourselves. What do we do with it? Surely it should be easy to make change happen now, right? Well, let's take a moment to talk about change.

Change can be incredibly hard and take a long time; it can also be super easy and happen immediately! Both of those statements are true, and so is everything in between. Each of us has our own special and unique relationship to change. In work, whether as a coach, mentor or consultant, I speak with people about change all the time. It becomes part of my everyday vocabulary and the subject of most conversations. I work with people who get stuck, who crave change, who want to be in a different situation. I offer them space to think, reflect, analyse and plan. I make it look easy.

Why then, when I go for my morning swim at the gym, do I lose my mind if I get to the changing room to find that someone is using my locker? In truth, it is not technically my locker, I just like 286. So, I have used it nearly every day for several years. It messes up my day if someone forces me to change, especially at 7am. It isn't just long-standing relationships like the unbreakable bond between a man and a small cupboard either. It could be that this is some primordial territorial thing, or perhaps I get weirdly attached to lockers – really, though, I think it's more about the fact that I have to make a change when I don't want to.

Change, when we approach it with energy and determination, feels so powerful and liberating. When it is imposed, it can be devastating, because we are at heart irrational, emotional, illogical creatures who get weirdly attached to people, places and things. Even change that is seemingly positive comes with loss. The great new job might mean leaving a team of people you feel totally comfortable in. The move to a better house in another area could leave you feeling disconnected from friends and neighbours. Getting married could put an end to your feelings of freedom. Every positive change is accompanied by a touch of loss, even if it is tiny. That's why when I say that change is incredibly hard and super easy, both are true.

CONTEMPLATING CHANGE

- What is your relationship with change like?
- Do you welcome it or reject it?
- Does the idea of sameness feel comforting or terrifying?
- When do you know you are ready to make a change happen?
- What are your recollections of times you tried to make a change and failed gloriously?
- What have you learned about yourself and change throughout your life?
- What do you want to change in your life right now?

You can't change other people, only yourself. If you take radical, unconditional self-acceptance and mixed it with life-altering transformational change in the crucible of your queer wholeness, you have the potential for understanding the power that is available to you already, inside you, that nobody can ever take away.

Change involves beginnings, middles and endings. To let change happen, we have to let something go.

- How are you with endings?
- Do you prefer beginnings? If so, why?
- What's it like in the middle when things are just chugging along?

We don't always do endings very well. We move on. There is a place of healthy closure somewhere between keyhole surgery and open, weeping wounds. Ending well, deliberately, should be available to us as an option. The big ending we all face is death, which for me now feels, if not close, at least visible on the horizon.

I have a fantasy, like most people, of a peaceful death where I drift off to sleep having completed my journey on Earth with everything ticked off my to-do list and a heart full of love. It will, of course, be messier than that. When my mum died, she was alone in her flat and was discovered by a family member who was worried they hadn't heard from her that morning. She died alone, on the floor, where she lay for maybe a day before she was found. I contrast this to my experience of her growing up. My mum was the life of any party. She was outgoing, kind, warm and magnetic. People loved being around her, up to a certain point. Sober, she was clear-eyed and hard-working. Drunk, she was unrecognizable. Over time, she alienated herself from everyone close to her, one by one, falling like dominoes. I lost contact with her two years before her death, only hearing stories of her from others who witnessed her increasingly problematic behaviour. I don't remember our last conversation, it was probably terrible, and at the time I had no idea it would be the final one. It's impossible for me to know how my mum felt in the days leading up to her death. I can't imagine she was happy. She was alone, lost and desperately ill. She died at the open, weeping wound end of the death continuum, as so many people who are lost to addiction do.

That is not my story. Not my future. Firing myself out of my uncomfortable zone – Aberdeen – and into a new life propelled me toward an adventure I could never have imagined possible. In middle age, I can appreciate the mistakes, learn from the bad choices and consider what I do next with my life. Taking myself through The Queer Wholeness Method has revealed this about my wholeness.

I got to the place I am despite, and sometimes because of, changes in societal attitudes toward homosexuality that began in my childhood and continue through today. I grew up somehow understanding that my queerness was not the problem, other people were. I was able to recognize that sometimes it was not their fault and forgive them anyway. I can also forgive myself for the lies they told me that I believed.

I explored my experiences with shame, belonging, meaning, legacy and pleasure. The stories I reminded myself of opened windows to the moments that shaped me in my younger days that still show up today. The parts of my wholeness that still feel fractured include:

- Hidden shame I still carry about fancying men
- The stories of predators, dangerous promiscuity and other lies I believed
- My futile search for one single meaning of life, and the liberation of knowing I can have many
- The ambivalence I feel about belonging, except to my husband, which itself will lead to loss
- My struggle with legacy, walking the tightrope of changing the world or being forgotten
- The difficult relationship I still have with pleasure, rooted in fear of AIDS and others' judgement

As revealed in Part II, working through The Queer Wholeness Method helped me discover new knowledge about my whole. Here is a summary of what I learned:

> To be where I would like it to be, my self needs to invite my whole to get closer. My self needs to move around it, explore it. My whole wants to be understood, but it can't be properly known until it is examined further. My self knows where my whole is. There's a connection. I would like it to be even better.
>
> I discovered that there are still many hidden parts that I have not felt ready to look at. My wholeness revealed that by showing myself those hidden parts, I can understand myself better, that I may then show those parts to others, so they may feel able to look at their own.
>
> My wholeness is a rich tapestry of experiences and information. It's a dynamic landscape, alive with difference that creates the potential for life. It reveals my past but not my future, grounding me in the present.
>
> I can increase the depth, intensity or complexity of my whole by being bold in my alienness, showing my rainbow colours vividly, shining a positive light and holding space for the many possibilities that can emerge when I take myself deeper.
>
> My wholeness revealed that my queerness is power, light, magical, ancient, art. It showed me that I am nature, in nature. Everything about me is natural and nothing about me needs to change unless I want it to.
>
> The message I need to take, to myself and others, is one of acceptance.

That is the teaching I have gleaned from my Queer Wholeness. So, what might I do with that? For each of the themes I identified, I can apply the teaching of my whole.

The next step in our journey is to make a commitment to ourselves by writing a Queer Midlife Manifesto on how to turn those ideas into action.

I'm attracted by the idea of a manifesto because it feels quite punk. A good manifesto should act like a call to action. It ignites excitement and creates energy. That's the spirit I want to bring into the act of creating The Queer Midlife Manifesto – what will you bring to yours?

THE QUEER MIDLIFE MANIFESTO

> "My wish is that I always feel loved. And safe, I think, because that hasn't always been the case."
>
> – PAULA (AGE REDACTED)

The definition of manifesto is "a declaration of aims, intentions, motivations, values and views for how to be".

At this point in our process together, we can make a commitment to ourselves, and others, on how we want to live the rest of our lives. Or maybe just how we would like to be today. There are traditional methods of doing this, such as setting objectives, but they are pretty basic. They don't inspire imagination, and I believe that queer people are entitled to dream as bigly as possible. Instead of objectives, I invite you to create your own Queer Midlife Manifesto.

A manifesto is a written statement that we can use to clarify our goals to ourselves and communicate them to others. Writing a manifesto involves focusing on something we are passionate about, through which we can outline our beliefs. We can explain how our beliefs contribute to the bigger picture and make recommendations for changes that align with our goals, beliefs and behaviours.

A manifesto begins with an introduction to ourselves, a core message and a plan that inspires action.

Of course, you can use any medium you wish to create your manifesto. Express it as a piece of dance. Make a painting. Sculpt it from clay. Create a collage from pieces cut from magazines. I like to use words and then read them out loud, as if casting a spell. After all, there is magic in my Queer Midlife Manifesto.

Here are some tips for creating yours:

- Keep the language rooted in yourself. **Use "me" / "I"** when making your declarations.
- Lean into the possibility that **nobody ever needs to see your manifesto** except you and relish the freedom of expression that offers.
- Allow yourself permission to make **big bold promises** and paint them with bright colours. Or **keep them small** and as perfectly formed as you feel they need to be.
- Aim for something that, if read out loud, is **no more than a minute long**. Record yourself reading your manifesto and listen back to it. Re-write any parts where you don't hear your passion oozing into your ears.
- **Imagine reading your manifesto to your younger or older self.** What parts would each of them most appreciate? What do you need to say to yourself right now?

MY MIDLIFE MANIFESTO

My name is Paul, and I am a middle-aged queer person. I am grateful that I have made it this far and that there is so much further to go. I am passionate about bringing hope to others, and myself, with the rock-solid understanding that my queerness is part of a deeply felt wholeness. This wholeness is my doorway to understanding that I do not need to change anything about my queerness. It is as ancient as nature itself. I believe that the magic and art contained within my queer wholeness can be used as a powerful force for change, both within myself and others. Demonstrating acceptance of myself and boldness in showing my rainbow colours will help me and others to shine. My wholeness invites me to look at the hidden parts of myself that may still be holding me back, and share those too with others. My wholeness asks me to take myself into a deeper exploration of pleasure.

I promise to myself that I will:

- Visit and revisit my wholeness regularly, reminding myself that it is available any time I need it
- Look for opportunities to make art that might help me explore the hidden parts of myself
- Explore more deeply, and as often as possible, how I might experience true pleasure
- Practise acceptance of myself until it starts to feel as natural as breathing
- Share my learning of the gift of queer wholeness with others and invite them to explore their own whole

I feel inspired to find ways to gently conform less and less to others' expectations of me, in service of finding unconditional and lasting freedom, for that is my inalienable queer right.

Now, it's your turn.

What is your Queer Midlife Manifesto?

. . . .

. . . .

. . . .

. . . .

. . . .

. . . .

. . . .

LIVING YOUR MIDLIFE MANIFESTO

> “I never told my dad before he died. That was probably my biggest regret in life. I told him when he was in his coffin, when I went to see him at the undertaker's. I'm not sure how much he was listening – he probably wasn't his most attentive. But I think I knew somewhere in my heart I had to tell him, even in those circumstances."
>
> – DUNCAN, 51

We have reached the end of this part of our work together. Maybe more might happen in the future, who can tell. Humans love to pretend we can predict what's coming – whether it's forecasting the weather, studying futurology or setting betting odds – but in truth we are just another species walking in nature, trying not to fall off a proverbial mountain. There is strength in knowing that the future is unknown and being okay with that.

MY REFLECTIONS

In following the tools in this book, I have learned so much about myself and hopefully changed as a result. I was offered the privilege of hearing other people's stories, too, which is an experience I have so much gratitude for. I discovered that there was something at the core of our collective knowing, our queer wholeness, that was available to us if we looked for it and treated it kindly. Sharing stories, and being listened to with generosity and love, is a source of incredible support to ourselves and others. I want to do more of that.

I have come to a place where I am trying to be less singular in my thinking. There is no such thing as a typical queer person. We have unlimited possibilities of who and what we might be. When we consider what might come next, I no longer believe in a unitary idea of future. It is plural for me now. My futures. That one extra "s" adds so many infinite options to the amount, type and range of futures that I might both encounter and create for myself. My queer futures are waiting to be made and discovered. Thinking that we have just one possible path is so confining. I want the option of everything and anything, so I can choose what is the best option for me, right now, which might be different tomorrow or next year or the next decade. The vastness of my futures are so expansive, particularly compared to what was possible for me in the past.

To truly embrace and face those futures, I need to bring closure to some elements of what I have already lived through. I might need to create some endings before new beginnings can flourish. Middle age gives me an opportunity to reflect on things that no longer serve me: beliefs, patterns, stories, friendships, behaviours. Middle age is the perfect time to pause and re-assess what I want to take with me on the next stage of my journey. To do things out of happy, not habit. I also notice when there is a resistance to let go of particular things. For example, take those old friendships that fall into routine sameness. While they may have been full of energy and life at the start, they can begin to feel circular and dry. It does not mean I should necessarily let them go, but if I ask whether or not they align with my queer wholeness, my need to accept and celebrate myself, do they still fit? Attachment comes in many forms and not all of it is healthy.

I hope I have a long and happy life, which as a child never felt possible. The questions I face now are different ones:

- How do I stay healthy for as long as I can?
- How do I support the people I love as we encounter loss and setbacks?
- What might I offer myself and those close to me that could help us navigate what may, in fact, be the hardest part of the climb that is yet to come?

I have reached the summit of Mount Midlife, but standing here at the top means I can now see all of the mountains ahead of me. I'm excited that I get to climb those too, but one of them will be my last. At some point, I will have to face it, but there is still a lot of life to live before then.

EVER-CHANGING

So, where are we now? At this age, I thought I would be done with change. When I was younger, if I had ever been able to imagine myself at 50, I would have pictured a man with grey hair and a walking stick, living a contented and simple life. Thankfully, it didn't quite turn out like that. I am at a point, hopefully in the middle of my life, where newness feels possible. I recognize that not everything is possible. I don't believe in the kind of toxic positivity that says you can do anything you want to in life. Try telling that to a gay kid growing up in Kuwait. What I am convinced of, though, is that we have the potential to change what we can, if the conditions are supportive for us to do so. Outside forces can have a huge impact on us as queer people, and we should take comfort from – and maybe even celebrate – the fact that we are still here and still queer. The answer to *now what?* is up to us.

QUESTIONS TO PONDER

What's next for you?

What did you want at the start?

What have you learned about yourself?

Where are you now?

What might you do?

AN END OF A BEGINNING FOR THE EMERGING ELDERS

"I am the person who I am largely because of being gay. It's something to celebrate."

– ROBIN, 46

In various cultures around the world, elders are celebrated and revered as the wise people of the community. China has laws that require children to care for elderly parents. Families in South Asian, Latin American and many African cultures respect and admire the wisdom and knowledge their elders and ancestors pass on. Northern European and American societies have a more problematic relationship to our forebears. They are often seen as a burden or of decreasing use to society. Instead of taking their place at the heart of our communities, older people can be isolated, lonely and ignored.

Queer culture particularly struggles with the idea of ageing, possibly because we have few examples of positive, aspirational, healthy older role models. Older people in our communities have higher rates of depression and anxiety than the wider population, with few organizations tailored to meet their needs. Many over-50s still expect discrimination and stigma based on our sexuality and have particular concerns about care needs in later life. Within our community, there are common myths about being "old" at 25, which may once have been the case if life expectancy was short, but despite so much around us changing for the better, the stigma attached to ageing in the queer community is strong and present. We're still trying to play by the rules other people set for us. What if we had the chance to re-write those rules and play the game of life our way?

PLAYING THE GAME OF QUEER LIFE

> "I really enjoy sharing sex with my friends. It's connection in a way that I appreciate and enjoy."
>
> – RO, 40

A few years back, when our nieces were small, they wanted to play a board game with their uncles. They chose The Game of Life, which I had never seen before. As an only child, there wasn't much point in having board games, so I stuck to books instead. For others who may not know of this specific game, it's a standard board game in which your aim is to make the most money as you travel from early adulthood through to retirement. Whoever retires with the most cash, wins. There are blue pegs and pink pegs to represent people. You get money for going to university, getting a job, getting married and having children. The simple message is that to play The Game of Life, you must be straight. As I worked out what was happening, I began to get grumpy. I told our nieces that, actually, there are different ways to play this game. You can still be happy if you're not married. You might marry another girl, or you could have a boy and a girl in your marriage. You don't have to have children. You get the picture. Our youngest niece said she didn't want to play anymore, started to cry and told her mum I was ruining all the fun. That's the thing about playing a different game of life (in real life): it ruins the fun for people who benefit from playing the game. If they can see that we are able to still finish the game happy, regardless of how much money we have acquired, it drives them a little bit mad. Changing the rules of the game is hard, though. People stop playing when they realize you don't want to have their kind of fun. I also wonder if we have to play the game at all. What if we created our own version of the game? What might that look like? Here's my version:

- End the game as the kindest, most compassionate person you can become.
- Leave no physical clutter behind because anything you have accumulated will be given to charity and nobody else wants it anyway.
- Collect points every time you make someone's life a little better.
- Bonus points for inventing new forms of relationship models!
- Get extra turns if your life contributes to the health instead of the destruction of the planet.

PRIVILEGE AND PERSPECTIVE

Getting older provokes responses from everyone. No one, regardless of their sexuality, really likes to age. In our community, when telling people I was writing a book for middle-aged queers, many of the folk I spoke to clutched their invisible pearls in shock. "I'm not middle-aged, am I?" they'd ask. Technically, the definition of midlife is the period from 40 to 60, so if they fit into that bracket then I replied, "Yes, you're middle-aged." Nobody who got that response thanked me for it.

Society has always, and will always, favour the young. Whether it be ancient Greek sculpture or new-season ASOS, the inspiration will always come from 18–35s. The golden demographic. They make marketing people moist. If we look at it through a simplistic capitalist lens, of course, they're seen as the top of the pops. As I write this, young people are out there, being seen, showing off, taking selfies and making TikToks. Brands want them to be wearing their stuff and buying their shit so other young people will feel compelled to buy their stuff and wear their shit.

In midlife, we do have certain privileges. People might listen to us more. We might have more power. There are definitely benefits to ageing. Middle-aged people – and perhaps this is a sweeping generalization based purely on myself – stay at home more. We maybe have a little more money.

Of course, there are benefits to being young, and I remember some of them well. Pulling an all-nighter, hand-writing university assignments 12 hours before the submission deadline. Drinking until the early hours of the morning, eating a pasty from the petrol station, thinking, *No point sleeping now*, and then going straight to work looking and feeling like a car ran over me in same petrol station. Being able to masturbate more than once a day – or, let's be honest, week.

Youth is totally wasted on the young, which is what should happen. No young person deserves wisdom. They wouldn't know what to do with it anyway. Youth should be the space of stupidity, frivolity and mistakes. I hate the question "What do you wish you'd known when you were younger?" because it implies that I know anything better now. Younger me would have told older time-travelling me to fuck off, because he's old and judges me for eating petrol-station pasties.

The process of ageing does have its drawbacks, like the ever-looming spectacle of death, but mostly the benefits outweigh the losses. My friend Dan, 29, who works in a law firm doing something I don't understand, was reflecting on his life so far and wondering what the future might hold. "I'm looking forward to getting the keys to the third floor," he said, which I took to mean he was getting some promotion at work. What he actually meant was that turning 30 involved going up a decade, to a new level in the building of his life. He said a friend of his introduced him to the concept and said, "Wait till you get to the fourth floor, the hand soap is amazing," which is true.

I loved this image of ascending through the floors as we age. It's so much nicer than racing downhill fast, slumped over or going tits-up – all kinds of descriptions of ageing that, while funny, imply generally bad things. I prefer to see myself luxuriating on the fifth floor, to which I was recently given the keys. There's more perspective than I was afforded on the lower levels.

These middle floors, four to six, they hold a lot of meaning. We've lived lives and collected stories that fill our shelves. Some of the people we loved are not in the building anymore, but they still take up space in our hearts. A lot of queer folk never made it past the first or second floor, so I feel lucky to be up here taking in the view.

LIVING OUR MIDLIFE TRUTH

Midlife can be a minefield for queer folk. We encounter some of the same huge changes as our straight friends – career shifts, divorce, teenagers and routine existential crises – but we do it without a manual. Our queer ancestors had their own unique challenges to face, but many of them didn't make it this far, and their wisdom was lost. So, we are the midlife queers, the ones without a map. It's up to us to make our own. In a time of escalating negativity toward us, we must fight back by living our most joyful, vivid, visible queer lives, knowing that our wholeness is our superpower.

At various times in our lives – and sometimes in the space of one day – we might like, love, lust and loathe different aspects of our selves. Sometimes, it's easier to look away from the facets of ourselves that don't shine as brightly as the others. We are all changing all the time, and this is one of the greatest gifts of our humanity. Also, it's fine to want things to stay the same when it's going well. Our ability to ride the pendulum as it swings between change and stability is both a challenge as well as an opportunity. The path is ours to walk.

FACE THE WIND

“I’m suddenly realizing that I’m old and my voice has every right to be heard, if not more, about things that directly affect my life. These little clowns need to back the fuck up and start listening.”

– NICK, 45

What do you want to change in the world?

If I were to describe what motivates me, propels me forward, drives me, two words immediately come clearly into mind: hope and rage. They may seem like an odd pair, but like Bert and Ernie, they're actually much closer than we have been led to believe.

The stems of hope and rage both have their roots planted in the same soil that fostered the growth of the most powerful, effective and impactful people who ever danced across the face of the earth. Their passion for change and refusal to accept the status quo burst from them and fertilized the ground that supports us all. Our feet are held firm by the energy of greatness given to the world with generosity, grace and general badass-ness of those who pushed past anyone who stood in their way, refusing to go quietly into the night. Don't get me wrong: I am a fair-weather activist. I have no right to compare myself to any of the incredible changemakers who put their lives and freedoms at risk while I watched from the sidelines. Protesting as a 19-year-old student was easy; doing it as a 52-year-old with a business, husband, friends, family, bills, household responsibilities ... it's a lot. I never feel like I am doing enough.

SPARKS OF HOPE

My friend Kath curated an online exhibition during the Covid-19 pandemic when we were all divided, scared and isolated. She invited participants to create work that represented how we wanted the future to look once we returned to normal, whatever that was. I am not an artist, and the thought of being creative in that way filled me with dread, but I knew I wanted to make something that spoke to the resurgence of bigotry, racism and hatred that had been simmering and then reached boiling point after the murder of George Floyd.

I created a piece called "Love Bombs" – painted eggs filled with glitter, each containing a word: "racism", "homophobia", "transphobia", "sexism", "hatred". I made a box for the eggs with instructions for their use.

The purpose of the eggs was not to be looked at, but to be thrown. With Dan as my artist's assistant – he said artistic director, but that's fine – we went outside to film the piece. I threw the eggs against the wall of a nearby building, casting out the hatred and watching the dark bombs explode with colourful glitter on impact. It was cathartic, like casting a spell for hope. I thought to myself, maybe this is what activism is like.

Inside, it felt performative. I knew I was making this art to be featured in an exhibition. We filmed it with nobody nearby. Dan made me bring a dustpan and brush to clean the mess up afterwards. It was a very sanitized version of disturbing the peace. We left no trace of our activism. As I said, I never feel like I am doing enough.

When the flames of fear and bigotry rise higher, we have choices to make. Our decisions on how we participate are personal, private and rarely simple. Some of us will choose safety, hunkering down and hoping the storm passes. This is perfectly reasonable. Our survival should come first. The world needs all the queer people it can hold. Others will write blogs, share Instagram Reels or sign petitions – that's also fine. Some of us will join protest marches with homemade signs, chanting along with a little nervousness and self-consciousness. Others will organize the marches and shout the loudest. All of those are good. The only important thing is that we do something. Even if it is to choose to stay indoors and survive, it is still something. Doing nothing is no longer an option. Maybe it never was.

CHANNELLING RAGE FOR GOOD

Hope and rage co-exist like oil and water, never entirely changing the properties of the other, but providing enough tension to make something move. At my most hopeful, I can envision a world where our sexuality does not negatively impact our lives in any way. Unfortunately, that world will not happen in my lifetime, or maybe even the next. That's where the rage comes in.

How dare other humans tell us how we should or should not live, because of who we want to fuck? Particularly when it comes from a religious dogma, hiding behind the shield of an ancient text that somehow empowers ordinary people to be extraordinarily cruel to each other. I refuse to accept that this is the way things have to be any more. I will never accept intolerance. My life would be so much easier if I were indifferent. Apathetic. Turning my back. For many years I did. No more. As an emerging elder of this complex community, I must accept the flame being passed to me from those who held it for so long that it began to burn their hands. They deserve to enjoy their latter years, knowing they did all they could. It is our turn now.

SMALL ACTS OF RESISTANCE

At the intersection of hope and rage is mischief. We don't all have to chain ourselves to the gates of parliament to make a point. Small acts of queer resistance can be just as powerful, and maybe even fun. Deliberately misgendering a baby will show how quickly straight people believe in the importance of pronouns. Asking a straight man how long he and his husband have been together before apologizing and explaining how you didn't want to offend him by assuming he was heterosexual to show that no one's sexuality is preferable to another's. Just do something. Anything. A whole heap of something is better than shitloads of nothing.

Now that we've explored some of the events, emotions and experiences that brought us here, we can begin turning our attention to where we might like to go next. We might give ourselves permission to dream what a new future could look like if we change something – or some things – in our present.

QUESTIONS TO PONDER

What is your relationship to activism?

If you were to describe your inner emotional weather conditions right now, what are they?

Which of your emotional muscles needs a workout?

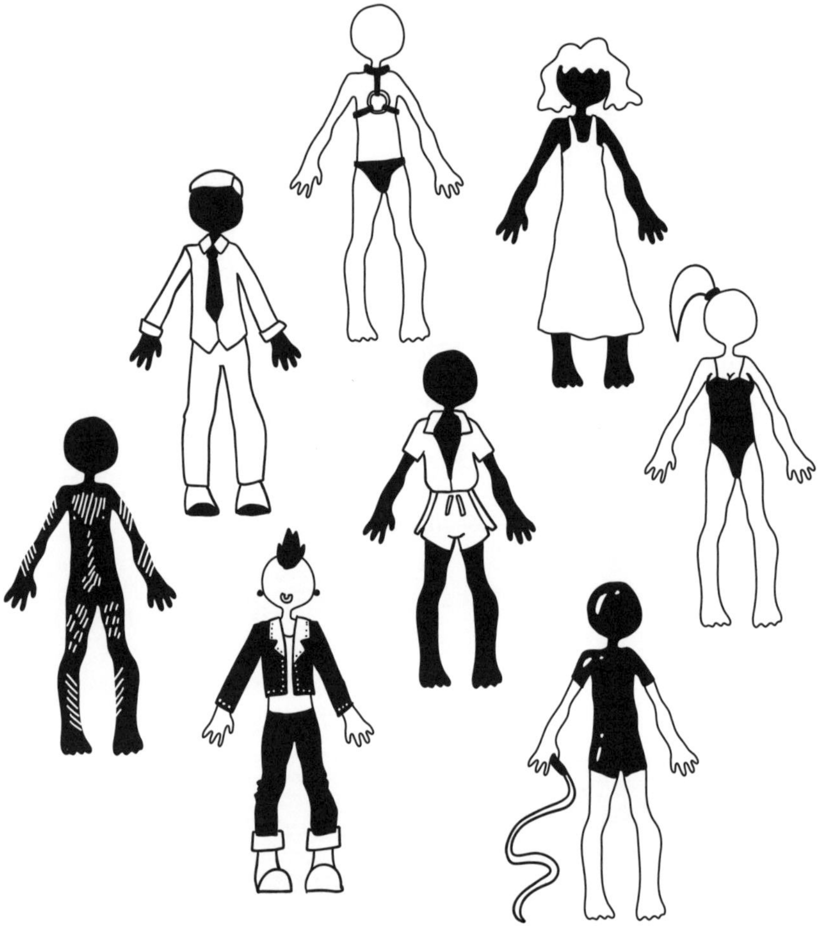

TOWARD QUEER COMMUNITY WHOLENESS

> Identifying as a non-binary person, having different gender pronouns, having a name that isn't like Brad or Joe, [...] for a lot of people, that's really confusing, and it's not a turn on at all."
>
> – XANDER, 42

What if we went beyond the individual, and created a Midlife Queer Community Manifesto? A series of conscious commitments to ourselves, our communities and our loved ones?

There is no need to agree with all of it, and you can change anything that doesn't completely resonate with you, but I think this list is quite comprehensive of what we can achieve in midlife for ourselves and each other.

The Midlife Queer Community Manifesto

Mid-way through our lives, we occupy space at the intersection of our pasts, presents and possible futures. This is our opportunity to celebrate how far we have come, and to redefine the idea of middle age in relation to queerness. This manifesto is a declaration of power. It describes our hopes, dreams and wishes, offering itself as a rallying cry to all who find themselves navigating the complex landscape of middle age with courage, resilience and a refusal to accept anything other than complete authenticity.

- We fully and unconditionally embrace our queerness.
- We redefine ageing with grace, power and dignity.
- We cultivate radical self-acceptance.
- We foster deep, meaningful, nourishing connections.
- We challenge invisibility and erasure through authentic self-expression.
- We advocate for inclusive, affirming spaces where we belong.
- We celebrate our changing bodies in all their unique forms.
- We effortlessly leave a legacy of love, peace and joy.
- We live deliberately and intentionally as emerging elders of our community.
- We reject anything that seeks to constrain us in the next phase of our lives.

This is an unwavering commitment to ourselves and our communities, a testament to the strength, resilience and beauty of living as middle-aged queer people. Together we will continue to learn, grow, nurture and uplift each other. We are still here, still queer and our stories are far from over.

WE ARE NOT ALONE

I spend my working days helping people and organizations that want to reinvent themselves in some way, and the common element of my work is that it is never done alone. Change is hard to do when nobody else is involved. In my field of work, we say that the group is the basic unit of change. People who come together for any purpose will either help or hinder each other's ability and capacity to change. This is true for families, friendships, work teams, communities, organizations, places, systems and the wider world. We are all connected, interdependent, social beings.

Reading a book is, in some ways, the opposite to that experience, although I hope that the relationship we've created through the exchange of my words and your brain has helped you feel a connection to me, my life and my work. Nonetheless, a book can't answer back. Books are unable to ask "Did you really mean that?" or "Are you sure that's the truth?"

Some people choose counselling or therapy, coaching or mentoring as a route to working with another person who is trained in methods that place you at the heart of the experience. You may be well acquainted with or want to explore those for yourself as part of your ongoing self-discovery. Less formally, we create and join groups of people – friends, colleagues, folk we share interests with – and build networks of mutual support and encouragement. Like everything, they can be tricky to navigate (maybe especially in middle-age, when some patterns feel more established and therefore harder to change), but they are a rich source of nourishment when they work well.

FINDING QUEER SPACES

For me, it has been important to find specifically queer spaces where I can be myself without having to explain who I am. I have enjoyed being with a gay men's meditation group, creating with a queer writers' group, working through stuff with a gay therapist and hosting a queer panel podcast. I visit a queer barber who takes care of my beard and a queer tattooist to make art on my body. These, of course, are not the only spaces in which I exist. I spend a lot of time with straight people at work, in the gym, on the Tube, in my family and friendships, and in all media consumption. The right balance for me is making sure I have specifically queer spaces for certain aspects of my life. They are important to me. I realize also how lucky I am to live in a place and time where I can have a queer barber and tattooist. Many of us live in places where access to queer spaces is not so readily available, if at all.

I encourage everyone reading this book to explore where they locate themselves in queer spaces. Do you have what you need or would you like something more, or different? Open a doorway into community that may not have been available before. You can connect to others in various ways:

- Use the #STILLHERESTILLQUEERNOWWHAT hashtag on social media as a way of finding ourselves through our posts. Share your Midlife Manifestos and make a public commitment to yourself.
- Create and/or join a virtual #STILLHERESTILLQUEERNOWWHAT book club meeting using the information later in the book.
- Show your whole with some #STILLHERESTILLQUEERNOWWHAT merchandise, posters and badges available from stillherestillqueernowwhat.com.
- Tell a friend about this book. Buy a copy for their next birthday. Leave a copy on a table in your local queer bar. Link to it from your social media profiles. Share the queer wholeness love.

QUESTIONS TO PONDER

What would you like to have happen next?

....

....

....

....

....

....

Without embarrassment or humility, what are the things you most deserve next?

....

....

....

....

....

....

....

What areas of your life need some attention?

....

....

....

....

....

....

....

CHANGE IN A TIME OF COMMUNITY COMPLEXITY

"As I'm getting older, I'm getting more and more angry. So, what I'm actually finding now is I'm actually more radical than I was when I was 28. I've been getting less tolerant. I'm starting to become much more of an activist again, which is something I never thought would happen. We need to stand up and be heard again."

– KEITH, 48

What major societal shifts have you lived through since you came out?

. . . .

. . . .

. . . .

. . . .

. . . .

. . . .

. . . .

. . . .

. . . .

As queer people, our ability to thrive depends significantly on where we are in the world. The global picture of LGBTQ+ rights is complex and varied. While we have undoubtedly seen huge progress in some places, there are significant – often life-limiting – challenges in others. It's reassuring to see that the trend in recent decades for countries protecting, and sometimes even celebrating, legal equality has brought freedoms and possibilities that were hard to imagine when I was a young kid. Many countries have introduced marriage equality and enforced anti-discrimination laws that help us to live more authentically as ourselves. It is, however, not the same around the world.

I was fortunate to meet one of my writing heroes, Armistead Maupin, a few years ago. I asked him what kept him fuelled to keep fighting for our rights and he said, "It's not okay until it's okay for everyone, everywhere." It was a humbling moment. There are still countries where queer people face legal and social persecution, unable to be who they are without life-changing consequences.

THE TIMES ARE A CHANGING

This regression to bad old days is not just downright dangerous to our safety, but it's difficult to navigate as a middle-aged queer person. I've noticed recently that I'm beginning to edge into a different demographic, and that I'm becoming part of history. I used to joke that I came out so long ago that I did it through the medium of cave-painting, but I actually had two experiences recently that made me feel like an actual fossil.

I was giving a talk at a networking event for young LGBTQ+ professionals. Once the talks were done and the wine was flowing, people came over to chat and ask questions. One amazing person asked the most beautiful questions. The first was "Has your queerness ever been a barrier to your career?" (short answer: no, I think it's my superpower), and the next question was "Why are you still putting yourself out there waving the LGBTQ+ flag?" I said it started when, as a student in the early '90s, I was literally on the streets waving a flag in protests where we were trying to get the age of consent for gay men reduced from 21 to 16. When I'd finished my little rant, the person who asked the question looked surprised and said, "The age of consent was 21? I didn't know that." I felt so happy that this person had never lived through a time when they didn't have pretty much the same rights as heterosexuals, but I wondered why they didn't know about our history.

Try telling a young queer person that there used to be a section in the *Pink Paper* (a physical kind of website) where you could post a personal advert in the classified section: men seeking men. If I saw someone who made themselves sound interesting in under 20 words, I could write a letter, enclose a photo and send it to the newspaper offices, who would forward it to the person who placed the ad. They might write back, offering a phone number. The time from reading the ad to speaking on the phone could take up to three months. Nowadays, people send a series of angry question marks if you don't reply to them on Grindr within three seconds.

The first time I saw an erect penis aimed at me – marketing-wise, not physically – was in *Zipper* magazine, which I bought in a sex shop in Soho and had to make last for at least six months. Now, I can find anything I want on PornHub, clicking endlessly through the list, searching for the perfect scene. There's just so much more choice than before. Everything is available.

As a community, we've gone from gay and lesbian to LGBTQIA2S+ in what feels like the blink of an eye. Conversations about intersectionality, identity and fluidity have so much more nuance than the "are you a poof?" question of my youth. Thankfully, we also understand a lot more about neuroplasticity than before. It is possible for an old dog to learn new tricks. It always was. Getting older is no excuse for resisting change, but the pace and depth of change we're living in today can, at times, make me want to hide under my weighted blanket.

MOVING FORWARD, TOGETHER

It used to be us against them – gays against straights – behind clear battle lines of right and wrong. Now, it's us against them *and* ourselves, fighting each other about whether trans people should be included in our collective while the straights also pile in. If someone had called themselves a straight, gay-friendly feminist 20 years ago I would have felt safe in their presence. Now, I worry that they're going to get all TERF-y on me. We're in a time of smudged boundaries, where everyone believes they are right and can make up truths to justify their own positions. The answer isn't to go back, which so much of today's politics teases as the answer, but to go boldly forward into uncertainty, embracing the complexity of living because we can. I have the gift of being alive that many of my peers and most of my queer elders no longer enjoy. When my heart is pounding at bedtime because I can't reconcile my mortality, I have to tell myself that I am not dead yet. I have life to live, even if it's a little less than before and getting shorter every day. I am still here, and still queer.

In midlife, I'm starting to develop more compassion for myself and use the gift of memory and hindsight to understand why it feels so difficult to make sense of things. Yes, the world has changed almost beyond recognition in the space of my lifetime, but I can't shake off some of those analogue attitudes. The fear of being myself without consequence. The shame that still shows when I try expressing my sexual desires. The belief that the world would rather not have me in it if this is how I choose to live my life. I am a questioning person in a world obsessed with answers.

OUR COMPLEX WORLD

I believe that being queer has a lot to do with complexity theory – bear with me. Complexity theory is concerned with living systems, how things are interconnected and interdependent. Complex systems adapt to their environments and respond to provocations. Within complexity is the idea of non-linearity, that a small change can have huge effects, and emergence, where patterns form that either amplify or dissipate over time. Complexity theory says everything is fluid and unpredictable, constantly changing and evolving. If complexity theory makes your ears prick up, wait until you hear what quantum mechanics has to say about time.

In many ways, my simple, gay childhood self has grown up into a complex queer world. Making sense of the realities of life today is hard enough, much less when carrying baggage from the old days that constantly shouts in my ear about how terrible it is to be gay. It might explain how, as a kid, I would have one long sleep through the night, and now, in middle age, I need multiple naps. Growing up gay was hard. Growing old is too easy. I'm not necessarily interested in cryogenically freezing my body or keeping my brain alive in a jar post-death, although it's tempting just to see what happens next, but I want to look my middle age squarely in the eye and say, "We've got this." For however many years I have in front of me, I want to make them better than those behind. Living is not as simple as it used to be, but grappling with complexity is sexy.

It's important to acknowledge and recognize those who have our backs. Who are your people? Draw them here.

QUESTIONS TO PONDER

What do you make of the state of the present-day world for LGBTQ+ folk?

. . . .

. . . .

. . . .

. . . .

. . . .

. . . .

How do you imagine the future to look for the LGBTQ+ community?

. . . .

. . . .

. . . .

. . . .

. . . .

. . . .

. . . .

Where, or who, are your lighthouses in a storm?

. . . .

. . . .

. . . .

. . . .

. . . .

. . . .

. . . .

CHANGE STARTS HERE, AGAIN

> “I struggle with wanting more emotional connection and I wear my heart on my sleeve in that respect. It's frightening to be authentic because it feels like most people aren't ready for it."
>
> – ADAM, 44

It's such a cliché to say that the only constant is change, but there's a lot of truth in it. When I began thinking about this book, we were at the tail end of a toxic, long-term conservative government in the UK. The prevailing tone of any conversation about diversity, gender and difference was increasingly bold and hostile. We were in the height of the so-called culture wars. Then the government changed, and while I looked at the incoming administration through half-closed eyes, suspicious of their intentions, it gave me the opportunity to exhale slightly. Hearing a politician say they would no longer indulge the narrative of culture wars was so freeing. Kamala Harris declared she was running for president, and again, my eyes were half-closed with some suspicion about her track record, but her election message seemed so hopeful: "We're not going back." Strangely, I began to get nervous that my book wasn't needed. What if suddenly everything got better again? Maybe I was just in the middle of a particularly bad era that made me believe the book was essential.

Now the book is out in the world just as I have become more fearful than ever before. The UK government continues to endorse a destructive perspective on trans rights. Donald Trump is back in the White House. Social media has taken a sharp nosedive into right-wing ideology. Part of me feels slightly embarrassed to say this, but it has made me feel a certain kind of aliveness. We have something to fight against, not just whispers and coded dog-whistle conversations. We are hearing actual, real people say harmful and dangerous things about us again. I'm not happy that this is the case, yet something has awoken in me as I finished writing this book. There have been times during the writing process when I felt exhausted, wondering if I could finish it.

I ran my first marathon in 2012, and one of the best pieces of advice I was given was to check who was next to me as I was about to cross the finish line because that's who will be in the photo you'll always remember. I am by no means an athlete and spent most of the marathon being overtaken. Then, the moment came when I turned the corner and saw the finish line ahead. I had cried several times during the race, and despite the incredible tiredness, I steeled myself to make sure that I finished strong. It didn't actually matter who was there with me as I crossed the line, as we had all achieved something pretty spectacular. Energy suddenly appeared in my legs after 26 miles, and I crossed the line smiling, walked to the pub and felt fresh as a daisy. I'm feeling something similar today. This is not the end of the book. It is the beginning of a whole new race. The terrain is more treacherous, and fewer people are cheering us on from the sidelines. Some are actively booing. We are running the race together until the time when our individual finish line is crossed. I want to run this next leg the best way I can, supporting each other along the way as we celebrate reaching the end of this incredible adventure. Until the day comes when I cross my own finish line, I want to walk through the world connected to my queer wholeness, remembering that it is my power.

Beautifully, my wholeness is not finite. It is unlimited and rechargeable. I can top it up from a hug with an old friend. I can power myself up with a walk by Canal Street in Manchester. Energy can be replenished by reading a poem from a queer writer or listening to my favourite song by a queer artist for the 429th time in a row.

It's another cliché that you come into this world alone and you die alone. I've never believed that to be the case. I was not alone when I was born. I have lived my life in the company of incredible people, and as I face this next phase of my life, I hope I continue to connect with, love and celebrate more and more queer people. Those no longer with us in person are still carried in my heart. I will not die alone. I hope that moment is a long way in the distance because I want to celebrate that, for now, I'm still here, I am still queer, and I will be grateful for that until I take my last queer breath.

How will you top up your queer wholeness?

GRATITUDE

> “I wish for a revolution of acceptance that would reach far beyond the notion of sexuality. To see a way for us to centre belonging for everybody. Acceptance of everyone.”
>
> – RICHARD, 41

Thank you for picking this book up. Maybe you bought it, borrowed it, stole it or listened to it. However it happened, you have come to this place. I wish to express gratitude to you. It hasn’t always been easy for me to be grateful. I have no wish to grow old gracefully, but I hope I can do it gratefully.

My meditation app, like a stuck record on my phone, tells me constantly that the answer to pretty much everything is gratitude. The annoying thing is, it does work. On a particularly grumpy morning on holiday, I stood looking at the ocean with the sun in my face and sand between my toes. I wanted to roar into the waves, hoping they would carry all my fear and worries away. I didn’t, of course, because there were others on the beach and I cared too much about what they might think of me, so I held it in and stomped along the sand. “Why don’t you do a walking meditation?” my husband suggested, which, in hindsight, may just have been a smart way of diffusing my mood away from him. I put my headphones on and fired up Insight Timer, finding a session called Sacred Walk. It was 30 minutes long, and by minute 12, I could have wept. The calming Canadian voice in my ears reminded me that I was enough, I was worthy, I was powerful, I had a purpose and I had something to offer the world. She encouraged me to be grateful for every experience that had brought me to this moment and thank them for the gifts they offered. I felt my steps on the beach become lighter and softer.

I breathed more deeply. I was walking along a beach, in the sunshine, a 50-year-old gay man, running my own business, writing a book, blessed with amazing friends and a 25-year relationship with a man I am still so deeply in love with. Fuck me. How did that all happen? The gratitude meditation told me none of it was accidental. I had made it all work out this way. She invited me to feel the glow of love in my heart and beam it into the world. I imagined a big rainbow beam of light shooting from my chest, covering the sand and the sea and the people in amazing, beautiful love. Quite the contrast from the belly full of dragon fire I had arrived on the beach with. Same energy, different intention.

What makes it so hard for me to feel gratitude as easily as I feel frustration? It sounds a little trite to me, but the word that keeps coming up is "injustice". I am very motivated by fairness. I follow rules. I do my best. I try to help others. I like to talk people up. I am an unapologetic fanboy of the things I love. I am loyal and dependable. When I see others behaving in ways that feel unjust, it boils my piss. I hate people who hate people.

Ultimately, we are all just grains of sand on that beach, being moved by the wind and the waves, sometimes sparkling in the sunshine if we're lucky. We didn't ask to be born, but we were anyway. Let's be grateful for that.

What are you grateful for right now?

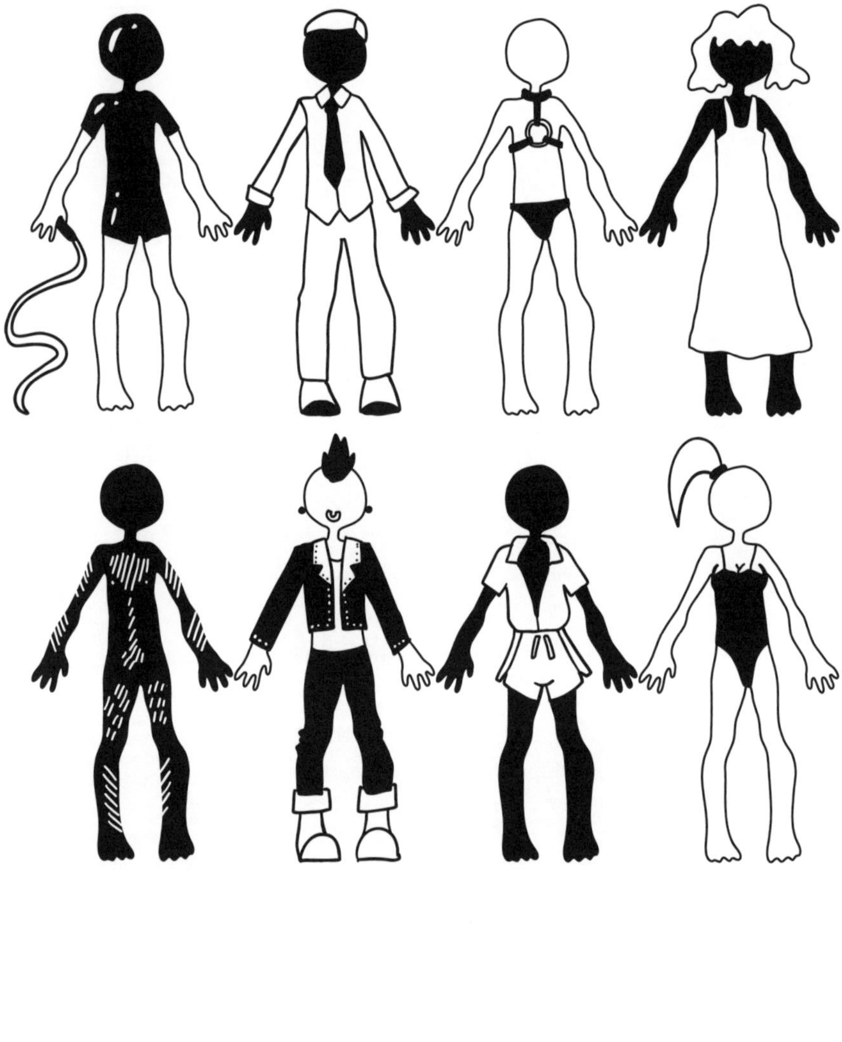

EPILOGUE

> “If you don’t actually do it now, actually make the change now, then when are you going to do it?”
>
> – STUART, 45

I didn’t plan on finishing my book today, it just happened. The signs were there though. I’d just spent an hour crying at the UK AIDS Memorial Quilt on display at London’s Tate Modern. Names of those lost too soon were read aloud as my face burned with tears of rage and sadness. All these people, gone. Most barely in their thirties.

Standing in this space of anger and pain I felt my pulse. My heart was beating fast with so much emotion. It was a great reminder of my aliveness. My blood still pumps. I have the gift of life denied to so many of those who would have become our queer elders, role models and mentors. As I finish with these final words, ready to send this love letter into the world, I celebrate everyone who came before us, the ones entering our elderhood and the younglings who might take inspiration from the paths we cleared for them, as those before me did with such passion and fire.

QUEER. WHOLE.

Change happens. Release yourself. It’s time for fresh skin. Inside us, every second, our cells are exploding. Newness is birthing visceral freedoms that can no longer be contained or controlled. As if they ever could.

Our sole task is to witness the emergence of the self that wishes to be here next. Let go of now. Answer the call. Shift shape. It is happening with or without you, so just enjoy the ride. Feel the intense vibration as the self you desire is delivered into ecstatic soil. There is patterning in process, echoes throughout eternity of the people you were and will be. The ultimate galactic gang-bang where everyone climaxes at the same time and the sky sighs with unharnessed joy.

Wholeness is yours. It always was.
Still here. Still queer. Now, take the world.

DR PAUL TAYLOR-PITT

RESOURCES

SUPPORT AND RESOURCES

Working on ourselves can stir things up. Don't go through it alone. There are people who can help.

UK SUPPORT, ADVICE AND RESOURCES

Mental health and emotional support

MindOut

A mental health service specifically for LGBTQ+ people, offering online chat support, mental health advocacy and group support sessions

mindout.org.uk

LGBT Foundation

Offers support for a wide range of mental health issues, including online and phone support, peer support and counselling

lgbt.foundation

QUEERWELL

A community-led mental health and wellness charity offering in-person and virtual spaces for connection

Queerwell.org.uk

Switchboard

A helpline staffed by LGBTQ+ volunteers, providing support, advice and information on a range of issues including coming out, loneliness and mental health

switchboard.lgbt

London Friend

London-based support for LGBTQ+ people dealing with addiction, mental health and loneliness; also offers counselling and social groups

londonfriend.org.uk

Mermaids

Charity and advocacy organization supporting trans, non-binary and gender-diverse children, young people and their families

mermaidsuk.org.uk

Samaritans

Offers 24/7 emotional support and a non-judgemental listening service to anyone – not just the LGBTQ+ community – which can be very helpful for individuals struggling with mental health

samaritans.org

Connection and community

Out and About

A social and support group for LGBTQ+ individuals over 50, providing safe spaces and events across the UK to meet and socialize

outinthecity.org

Gendered Intelligence

Trans-led and trans-involving charity that works to increase understandings of gender diversity and improve the lives of trans people

genderedintelligence.co.uk

Stonewall

A charity that works to ensure acceptance for LGBTQ+ people in society, providing resources, campaigns and guidance on many issues facing the LGBTQ+ community

stonewall.org.uk

Pride in Ageing by LGBT Foundation

A programme specifically designed to tackle issues related to ageing and being LGBTQ+, offering resources, events and advocacy for older LGBTQ+ individuals

lgbt.foundation/pride-in-ageing

Legal support and advice

Galop

An anti-violence charity that provides advice and support for LGBTQ+ people facing hate crimes, domestic violence and sexual abuse

galop.org.uk

Citizens Advice

Provides valuable legal and financial support to anyone; can refer LGBTQ+ individuals to specific resources for issues such as discrimination and housing

citizensadvice.org.uk

LGBT+ Domestic Abuse Helpline (run by Galop)

Offers confidential advice and support, specifically for LGBTQ+ people experiencing domestic abuse

galop.org.uk/domesticabuse

Health and wellbeing

Terrence Higgins Trust

A leading HIV and sexual health charity offering support, information and resources for LGBTQ+ individuals, particularly those living with or affected by HIV

tht.org.uk

The Beaumont Society

Support and advice specifically for the transgender community, providing safe spaces and support networks for trans and gender-diverse people

beaumontsociety.org.uk

Positively UK

Provides peer support, advocacy and information for people living with HIV, with a strong focus on creating supportive communities

positivelyuk.org

Support for queer people of colour

UK Black Pride

Promotes unity and inclusion for LGBTQ+ people of colour, offering events, resources and community networks

ukblackpride.org.uk

Naz

Provides sexual health and HIV support services for BAME communities, including culturally specific support for LGBTQ+ people of colour

naz.org.uk

Employment and financial support

Diversity Role Models

Provides LGBTQ+ role models in educational and workplace settings, creating a safer and more inclusive environment – particularly helpful for those in career transitions

diversityrolemodels.org

ACAS

Provides anyone with legal advice and support regarding employment rights and discrimination, which can benefit those in the LGBTQ+ community facing workplace issues

acas.org.uk

US SUPPORT, ADVICE AND RESOURCES

Mental health and emotional support

The Trevor Project

Provides 24/7 crisis intervention and suicide prevention services for LGBTQ+ youth, but also a valuable resource for individuals of all ages

thetrevorproject.org

SAGE (Services & Advocacy for GLBT Elders)

The largest national organization dedicated to improving the lives of LGBTQ+ older adults, offering services, advocacy and community-building resources

sageusa.org

LGBT National Help Center

Offers confidential peer-support, information and local resources through hotlines and online chat services for people of all ages in the LGBTQ+ community

lgbthotline.org

The National Queer and Trans Therapists of Color Network (NQTTCN)

Focuses on mental health resources and therapy access for queer and trans people of colour, and provides a directory of affirming therapists across the USA

nqttcn.com

The GLBT National Hotline

Provides free and confidential support, offering resources and information for LGBTQ+ individuals via phone or email

glbthotline.org

Connection and community

CenterLink

A network of more than 250 LGBTQ+ community centres across the USA, providing opportunities to connect with others and attend social events, and giving access to local resources and support services

lgbtcenters.org

PFLAG (Parents, Families, and Friends of Lesbians and Gays)

Provides support, education and advocacy for LGBTQ+ people and their families; local chapters across the USA offer group meetings and community events

pflag.org

Legal support and advocacy

Lambda Legal

A non-profit organization working for the civil rights of LGBTQ+ people and those living with HIV through legal representation, policy advocacy and public education

lambdalegal.org

The National LGBTQ Task Force

Advocates for LGBTQ+ rights through social justice initiatives and legal reform, and offers resources and guides on navigating legal challenges via their website

thetaskforce.org

Transgender Law Center

Advocates for the rights of transgender and gender-nonconforming individuals, offering resources and support to navigate legal systems

transgenderlawcenter.org

Out & Equal Workplace Advocates

Focuses on LGBTQ+ workplace equality, offering resources and support to navigate discrimination and create inclusive work environments

outandequal.org

Health and wellbeing

Fenway Health

A Boston-based LGBTQ+ health organization offering healthcare, mental health services and support programmes for LGBTQ+ people, with many resources available online

fenwayhealth.org

Callen-Lorde Community Health Center

Based in New York City and provides LGBTQ+-focused healthcare, including primary care, mental health support and sexual health services

callen-lorde.org

Planned Parenthood

Offers inclusive and affirming healthcare for LGBTQ+ people, including sexual health services, counselling and hormone therapy at many locations

plannedparenthood.org

AIDS United

A national organization dedicated to ending the HIV epidemic, providing advocacy, funding and resources for people living with or affected by HIV

aidsunited.org

Support for queer people of colour

The Audre Lorde Project

A community-organizing centre for LGBTQ+ people of colour, focusing on social and economic justice, advocacy and community building

alp.org

Black LGBTQIA+ Migrant Project (BLMP)

Offers support for Black LGBTQ+ migrants, including advocacy, community-building and health resources

blmp.org

GLMA (Health Professionals Advancing LGBTQ+ Equality)

Provides resources for LGBTQ+ people of colour seeking inclusive healthcare providers

glma.org

Employment, housing and financial assistance

The Ali Forney Center

Provides housing and support services for homeless LGBTQ+ youth and adults in New York City and beyond

aliforneycenter.org

National Center for Transgender Equality (NCTE)

Offers resources and advocacy for trans people facing issues like employment, housing discrimination and healthcare access

transequality.org

Point Foundation

Provides scholarships, mentorship and leadership training for LGBTQ+ individuals pursuing education or career development

pointfoundation.org

SUPPORT, ADVICE AND RESOURCES IN AUSTRALIA

Mental health and emotional support

Qlife

A national LGBTQ+ peer support and referral service available via phone or online chat; provides support for mental health, coming out, relationships and more

qlife.org.au

Switchboard Victoria

Offers a free and confidential support service for LGBTQ+ people, including peer support, suicide prevention and family violence support

switchboard.org.au

Beyond Blue

Provides mental health support to anyone, but has dedicated resources for LGBTQ+ people experiencing depression, anxiety or isolation

beyondblue.org.au

Black Rainbow

Supports the social and emotional wellbeing of Aboriginal and Torres Strait Islander LGBTQ+ people

blackrainbow.org.au

Connection and community

LGBTQ+ Health Australia (formerly the National LGBTI Health Alliance)

An umbrella organization for LGBTQ+ health and wellbeing services across the country, supporting mental health, social connection and aged care programmes

lgbtihealth.org.au

GRAI (GLBTI Rights in Ageing)

Focuses on improving the quality of life for LGBTQ+ elders, offering support, advocacy and programmes to combat isolation

grai.org.au

Older LGBTI Advisory Group (Rainbow Connection)

Provides programmes and events to connect older LGBTQ+ Australians with peers and community support networks

thorneharbour.org

Thorne Harbour Health (formerly Victorian AIDS Council)

Offers a range of health and wellbeing services, including counselling, social support groups and health education

thorneharbour.org

Legal support and advocacy

Equality Australia

Advocates for LGBTQ+ rights, offering legal advice, support and resources on issues such as discrimination and workplace equality

equalityaustralia.org.au

LGBTIQ+ Legal Service (Victoria)

Offers free and confidential legal advice and support for LGBTQ+ people facing discrimination, workplace issues or family law matters

lgbtiqlegal.org.au

Human Rights Law Centre (LGBTQ+ Rights)

Advocates for LGBTQ+ equality through legal action, policy reform and public campaigns

hrlc.org.au

Health and wellbeing

ACON

Provides HIV prevention, sexual health services and LGBTQ+ wellbeing programmes, as well as a dedicated programme for older LGBTQ+ individuals called the LOVE Project

acon.org.au

SHINE SA

Offers sexual health and wellbeing services for LGBTQ+ people, including counselling, health promotion and medical services

shinesa.org.au

Living Positive Victoria

Provides support, advocacy and peer networks for people living with HIV, including resources specifically for older adults

livingpositivevictoria.org.au

Twenty10

Offers housing, mental health and social support for LGBTQ+ people, particularly young and middle-aged adults based in Sydney

twenty10.org.au

Support for queer people of colour

Black Rainbow

Specifically supports Aboriginal and Torres Strait Islander LGBTQ+ people, focusing on mental health, social justice and suicide prevention

blackrainbow.org.au

Australian GLBTIQ Multicultural Council (AGMC)

Advocates for the needs of LGBTQ+ people from multicultural and multi-faith backgrounds; hosts events, provides resources and connects individuals to community groups

agmc.org.au

Employment and financial support

Pride in Diversity

Supports LGBTQ+ workplace inclusion by working with employers and employees to create affirming environments

prideinclusionprograms.com.au

WorkItOut

Offers career support and job-seeking assistance for LGBTQ+ individuals, particularly those in career transitions

Australian LGBTQ Inclusion Awards

Recognizes organizations committed to creating inclusive workplaces, providing resources for LGBTQ+ individuals seeking supportive employers

Housing and aged care

Rainbow Tick Accreditation (Quality Innovation Performance – QIP)

Assists aged-care providers and health services in becoming LGBTQ+ inclusive, helping individuals find affirming services

rainbowhealthaustralia.org.au

Switchboard's Out & About Program

Provides community visitors for LGBTQ+ people in aged care or who are socially isolated

switchboard.org.au

HAAG (Housing for the Aged Action Group)

Offers housing support for older LGBTQ+ people to ensure they can access safe and affirming accommodation

oldertenants.org.au

PAUL'S PICKS: BOOKS AND PODCASTS

BOOKS

Non-fiction books are easy to recommend, as the writers are telling their own story, which means my personal taste doesn't come into it. I chose these books because the writers and stories are powerful, honest and wonderful.

- *Maggie & Me* by Damian Barr
- *Pleasure Activism* by Adrienne Maree Brown
- *Trans Britain* by Christine Burns (ed.)
- *Logical Family: A Memoir* by Armistead Maupin
- *Help* by Simon Amstell
- Anything by David Sedaris – honestly, anything
- *Boys Keep Swinging* by Jake Shears
- *Modern Nature* by Derek Jarman
- *We Can Be Heroes* by Paul Burston
- *Ten Steps to Nanette* by Hannah Gadsby
- *The Book of Non-Binary Joy* by Ben Pechey
- *Breaking the Rainbow Ceiling* by Layla McCay
- *Thank You for Calling the Lesbian Line* by Elizabeth Lovatt
- *Outrage* by Ellen Jones
- *Amateur* by Thomas Page McBee
- *Between* by Gemma and Leo Telford
- *Pop Scars* by Anthony Kavanagh

Fiction books are harder to recommend because, like music, they reflect the taste of the reader. I hope that my taste in books is better than my terrible taste in music. Here are some of the books by queer authors that I have really enjoyed:

- *Bored Gay Werewolf* by Tony Santorella
- *A Taste of Iron and Gold* by Alexandra Rowland
- *Before I Go to Sleep* by S J Watson
- *Legends and Lattes* by Travis Baldree
- *Her Majesty's Secret Coven* by Juno Dawson
- *The Whale Tattoo* by Jon Ransom
- *Everything Not Saved* by N M J Coveney
- *Wolfsong* by T J Klune
- *Arthur and Teddy Are Coming Out* by Ryan Love
- *The Pharmacist* by Justin David
- *The Madonna of Bolton* by Matt Cain
- *Invisible Monsters* by Chuck Palahniuk
- *Isaac* by Curtis Garner
- *Human, Animal* by Seth Insua

PODCASTS

- Attitudes
- Lovett or Leave It
- Handsome
- Keep It
- Talk ART
- Gayish
- Pop Pantheon
- Pause...and Rewind with Neil Hudson-Basing

... AND THE PODCASTS I HAVE CREATED

- HOPECAST
- Exploring the Heart of Change
- Still Here! Still Queer! Now What? The Podcast!

BOOK CLUB QUESTIONS

There are, thankfully, many queer book groups, writers' groups, Pride events and podcasts where we can be part of a wider discussion about ourselves and our relationship to this work. If you are considering holding space for folk to talk about *Still Here! Still Queer! Now What?*, I offer you these suggestions with an understanding that you may already have your own process and skills for facilitating discussions in a perfectly brilliant way – that's great. I just want to make sure that we take care of ourselves and each other in spaces where we might be disclosing details that might make us feel exposed, vulnerable, excited, worried, hopeful or fearful. These guidelines can also be used by people who have never held a space like this before and would like to give it a try with this book.

Still Here! Still Queer! Now What? offers rich material for book group discussions. It's the first self-help – what I call "biblio-coaching" – book specifically aimed at middle-aged LGBTQ+ individuals, but its themes of identity, ageing, community and self-discovery resonate far beyond this demographic. Featuring this book in your group will provide an opportunity to explore diverse perspectives, challenge assumptions and foster deeper conversations about the universal human experience of navigating life's transitions.

This book is not just for middle-aged LGBTQ+ people; it's for anyone interested in personal growth and wellness, and in understanding the diverse ways in which people experience midlife. By choosing this book, your group can engage in a meaningful exploration of what it means to live authentically, build community and support one another through life's challenges.

DISCUSSION TOPICS

To help your book group dive into *Still Here! Still Queer! Now What?*, consider using the following discussion topics:

1. Universal themes of midlife

- How does the book's portrayal of midlife challenges and opportunities resonate with your own experiences, regardless of sexual orientation or gender identity?
- What are the common fears and hopes associated with ageing that the book addresses? How do these reflect broader societal attitudes?

2. Identity and self-acceptance

- Discuss the book's exploration of identity and self-acceptance. How do the concepts of queerness and midlife intersect in the narratives shared?
- How does the book challenge or reinforce your understanding of what it means to live authentically?

3. Community and belonging

- The book emphasizes the importance of community and connection. How do these themes play out in the book, particularly in the author's stories?

- In what ways can your own communities become more inclusive and supportive of diverse identities and experiences?

4. Practical strategies for wellness

- What practical advice or strategies from the book stood out to you? How might these be applicable to people beyond the LGBTQ+ community?

- Discuss the importance of self-care, mental health and intentional living as presented in the book. How can these practices be integrated into daily life?

5. Broader social context

- The book touches on the social and historical context of ageing as a queer person. How does this context impact the author's life?

- What insights does the book offer about the ongoing struggles for visibility, equality and acceptance within the LGBTQ+ community? How are these relevant to wider societal conversations?

6. Bridging the gap between generations

- The book addresses the loss of an older generation of queer role models due to the AIDS crisis and other factors. How can younger and older generations within and outside the LGBTQ+ community support and learn from one another?

- Discuss ways in which the book encourages intergenerational dialogue and understanding.

PROMOTING INCLUSIVITY

To ensure that your book group understands that *Still Here! Still Queer! Now What?* is for everyone, consider these approaches:

- Highlight universal themes. Emphasize the book's exploration of universal themes like ageing, identity, self-acceptance and community, which are relevant to all readers, regardless of their background.

- Encourage diverse participation. Invite members from different age groups, backgrounds and identities to join the discussion. This will help create a richer conversation and demonstrate the book's broad appeal.

- Frame the book as an opportunity for learning. Position the book as a chance to learn about the experiences of a community that may be unfamiliar to some readers. Encourage members to approach the book with an open mind and a willingness to expand their understanding of diverse life experiences.

- Use inclusive language in promotions. When promoting the book discussion, use language that invites all readers to participate, regardless of whether they identify as LGBTQ+ or are in midlife. For example, you might say, "Join us for a discussion on the universal themes of identity, ageing and community, as we explore the groundbreaking book *Still Here! Still Queer! Now What?*"

- Create a welcoming environment. Ensure that your book group is a safe and welcoming space for all participants, where everyone feels comfortable sharing their thoughts and experiences.

RUNNING THE GROUP

Groups are funny things. People behave differently in groups than they do alone or with another person. We act in weird ways, say things we don't mean and go home wondering why we didn't talk about the thing we actually wanted to. So, I recommend you start by acknowledging that groups are strange yet wonderful spaces where we need to work out our own process for participation.

Consider the following when setting up your space:

- Who is invited and who is excluded?
- Do participants need to reserve their place or can they show up?
- Is there a minimum and maximum number for the group to run?
- Will the group meet only once, or is there a hope for more?
- Are participants expected to have read the book and completed The Queer Wholeness Method, or will you work through it together?
- What kind of space, materials, refreshments, facilities and resources do you need?
- If you are meeting in a physical place, is it accessible to everyone?
- If you are meeting virtually, how will you decide what platform to use?

At the start of a discussion group, you might invite participants to say what brought them to the space. There are some key areas that should be talked about before any of the work is done. These include agreeing:

- Start, finish and break times
- Confidentiality and honesty rules
- How the group will treat each other with respect

- Ways to create the best space to talk and listen without interruption
- How to demonstrate honouring the wisdom of the individual
- Strategies for including everyone's voices equally
- What to do if someone is sitting with strong feelings
- The boundaries of what the space is (and isn't) for

Finally, here are some ideas for conversation starters and questions for the discussion:

- How old are you, and what is that like?
- When did you first come out to yourself?
- What signals did you pick up when you were younger that gave cues you could (or couldn't) show your queerness?
- If you could have a conversation with your sexuality, what would it want to say to you about how it feels right now?
- What do you notice you feel more preoccupied with as you get older?
- Is there a wish you would like to make for yourself about how you'd like to live the rest of your life?
- What is the message you took from *Still Here! Still Queer! Now What?*
- Which aspects of the work held most significance or resonance for you?
- Were there parts of the process that had less impact?
- What did you learn about yourself that you didn't already know, and what did the book confirm for you?
- In what ways did the stories you tell yourself about yourself change as a result of the process?
- If you could tell your younger self about the method, what would you say? How about your older self?
- What conditions might you need around you in order for you to continue this work?

- Who could support you when things get tough? And when they're going great?
- What would you love to do with this new knowledge about yourself?
- Which aspects of your Queer Wholeness do you want to most celebrate?
- Where do you want or need to do more work on yourself?
- How might you find people to support you in those further inquiries?
- Which aspects of your Queer Midlife Manifesto are going well, and where might you need to change course?
- What support might you offer others?

Featuring *Still Here! Still Queer! Now What?* in your book group is an opportunity to engage in meaningful, thought-provoking discussions that transcend the boundaries of age and sexual orientation. By exploring the book's themes and encouraging inclusive conversations, your group can gain new insight into the diverse ways people navigate midlife and build a deeper understanding of the LGBTQ+ community. This book is a powerful tool for fostering empathy, connection and personal growth, making it a valuable addition to any book group's reading list.

References

Martha: The Life and Work of Martha Graham by Agnes De Mille. Random House, 1991.

Wholeness and the Implicate Order by David Bohm. Routledge Classics, 2002.

The Essential Jung: Selected Writings by Anthony Storr. Fontant Press, 1998.

Gestalt Therapy: Excitement and Growth in the Human Personality by Frederick S Perls. Gestalt Press, 1951.

The School of Life: An Emotional Education by Alain de Botton. Penguin, 2019.

The Nicomachean Ethics by Aristotle. Oxford World Classics, 2009.

Selected Writings by Thomas Aquinas. Penguin Classics, 1998.

The Wheel of Life as a Coaching Tool to Audit Life Priorities by Joan Swart, 2022.

Walk Through Walls: A Memoir by Marina Abramovic. Penguin, 2016.

The Varieties of Religious Experience: A Study in Human Nature by William James. Harvard University Press, 1902 (reprinted 1985).

An Essay Concerning Human Understanding by John Locke. Penguin Classics, 1997.

The Critique of Pure Reason by Immanuel Kant. Penguin Classics, 2007.

The Queer Child, or Growing Sideways in the Twentieth Century by Kathryn Bond Stockton. Duke University Press, 2009.

In a Queer Time and Place: Transgender Bodies, Subcultural Lives: 3 by Jack Halbertstam. NYU Press, 2005.

Gender Trouble: Feminism and the Subversion of Identity by Judith Butler. Routledge Classics, 2006.

Acknowledgements

Dan, thank you for showing me how to love. My eternal muse. The well of my inspiration ... is what my husband told me to say about him. Seriously, he made me write it down. Thing is, I couldn't have said it better myself. Dan, you are my world, my galaxy and my universe. You inspire me to do things that seem impossible because you show me how. Thank you for being utterly and beautifully yourself with me. While nobody will ever really know how funny you are, I get to see it every day and luxuriate in the bliss of being loved by you. What a gift! What joy! I love you.

Thank you to my parents for the love, lessons and encouragement to go for it. Special thanks to my second family, The Pitts and The Moyles, for making me your own.

My heart will always be with Nana, my safe place.

Words will never be enough to express my feelings of gratitude to the middle-aged queer folk who shared their stories with me.
An abundance of thanks (in no particular order) to: Gareth, Layla, Justin, Martin, Gordon, Abi, Lior, Adam, Gareth, Darren, Richard, Garvin, Duncan, Steve, Jon, Lizi, Paul, Nicholas, Paul, Ian, Lisa, Neil, Christianne, Andy, Mike S, Dave, Xander, Gordon, Bobbie, William, Jeremy, Dani, Sophie, Raga, Mike F, Robert, Mac, Paul, Dom, Phyll, Chloë, Liz, Karel, Sam, Phil, Matthew, Mike V, Aslan, Stuart, Johann, Eduardo, Keith, Grant, Gus, Craig, Paula, Johnny, Mark, Robin, Rey, Andy, Con, James, Paul, Ro, Neil, Steve, Chloë, Salim, Eva, Nick, Charlie and everyone who contributed and chose not to be named.

To the team who made this book possible, special thanks:
Abi at DHH Literary Agency, the best agent in the world, you believed I had a book in me before I did. You have the most incredible combination of pragmatic realism and enthusiastic dreaming. There is nobody I wanted to do this with other than you, and I am so grateful for the faith you had in me, and more importantly, this work. You are rainbow light personified.

Jane, Brooke, Sarah, Laura, Fi and the team at Jessica Kingsley Publishers, thank you for loving this book back to life and bringing it into the world. My gratitude is abundant!

Soraya, my OG editor who arrived in a burst of colour and energy that made me know you could give this book the love it needed – and by book, I also mean author. Thank you for making this dream real.

Andrea, thank you for the copy edit that made everything make more sense, although I still can't believe you didn't know about Madonna's near-death bacterial infection. I thought that was branded over our collective consciousness like the moon landing.

Neil H-B, your generosity and continued encouragement have meant the world to me. You are not just an incredible Tour Manager, you're also a badass fierce creative powerhouse and I am lucky to know you.

Anders, for illustrating the book so beautifully, squiggly, professionally and creatively. Thank you for getting it. You embody showing whole and queer excellence.

Ferg, creator of Propaganda, I love your sense of mischief and the playfulness you brought to the serious topic of phone box calling cards. Thank you for turning our bodies into art.

Steve Grolfe, thanks for the headshots. Finally a photo where I look and feel like myself.

My Book Squad, The First Readers Club, thank you for your careful and helpful feedback on the *Drag Race* Season 1 version of the book. You helped me remove the soft-focus filter.

The people who supported me through the writing process, there's a bit of each of you in these pages:
The Queer Writers' group who offered a safe haven for me to practise my craft. Caprice, Miss Kay, Erica, Avi, Marianne, Alex, Robin, Mo and everyone who came and is still to come.

Kate, Al, Lennox, Badri, Steve, Ted, Mary, Heather, David, Melissa, Ann-Marie, Emma, Sunil: The Catalan Crew, who stewarded and celebrated with me every day in a place of friendship, food and furry creatures.

We Create Space: Michael, Neil, Jon-Paul and the team, especially for the Soho House Sessions that opened a window into this work in the most beautiful way. Thank you for making space for the midlife queers. To the panel members who shared their stories, I loved every minute on stage with you.

Jo, thank you for our weekly focusing sessions that have helped me find myself again and again. You are part of this story at a cellular level.

Tomaso, for helping me reconnect to myself in ways I can never thank you enough for.

Kier, for the PT sessions that felt like physical and mental therapy during the writing process.

Damian, because you just get it like few others do. You have held a torch that has lit the path for me and I will always be grateful for yer big heart.

Steve, one day I aspire to sell millions of books like you have while at the same time staying humble and generous. Thank you for walking with me on this adventure.

Claire, thank for your wisdom in the wilderness. Look what appeared after the sandstorm!

My Learning set superstars: Dave, Jane, Deb, Caroline, Jeremy, Petra (Ronin Forever) Jae, David, Sanjay, Al, Maylis, Nicole and Dan.

My colleagues and trainers at The Somatic School, Nathan, Sam, Rachel and Craig, for making me a better coach and better person.

I am blessed with the most fucking wonderful friends in the world. I keep you apart because I want to have each and every one of you to myself, and I worry that you'll all like each other more than me and I'll be left out. In no particular order, and simply for the gratitude I have that you are in my life in some way, thank you to Andrea for decades of friendship (you are family like no other), Garry who brings out the best and worst in me (in the best ways), Davey for constantly inspiring me to create, Charlie (and Ronnie) for never giving up on me (and good belly rubs), Vilma for being the first person to say this book is needed and bringing precious joy, Sandi D for being a magical wonderful sage, Argyris for your boundless energy and encouragement, David K for showing me how to elevate my excellence, my token straight male friend Martin for the incredible conversations I can't have with anyone else, Dr Jack for being utterly perfectly yourself, Jonas for always bringing playful energy, The Sauna Sages (Paperboy David, Kev, Gordon, Beatles Paul) for sweaty and sweary chats, Steve for bringing your whole self to our friendship, Nicole for being bottled sunshine, Steve XOH for showing me how to be free, Chris, Sarah, Steph & Sandy for breaking out of workplace walls into wonderful friends, Woosh for embodying beautiful kindness, Rico for being my coolness role model, Trev for your generosity and super-connecting, Catherine for sharing the author journey including the scary parts, Diane for magically appearing when needed, Cip for your ability to rise, Nathaniel for always giving more, Nick for reminding me everything not saved is lost, Kav for showing your scars, Alexis for all your (blond) ambition, Alfredo for reminding me it's worth it, Thomas for the motivational personal podcasts, Layla for demonstrating how to conquer the world, Justin for unlimited generosity, and Katya for showing up with bundles of encouragement. I wish I could give each of you a page each with all the reasons I love you that couldn't fit here, but I'll end up writing a whole book about your brilliance, which is a great distraction from writing, and each of you at every step of the way have helped me to stay focused and believe that I can do this, so I'm sticking with that.

This book was conceived in a swimming pool in Gran Canaria before it grew into a fully formed life force in La Garigga de Castrelladal. It took shape in Copenhagen, grew wings in Cardiff and burst into flames in Manchester. The places where this book came to life became incredibly important, particularly when I was watched over by attentive and caring people. Having a safe space to think and write is priceless, so grazie mille to the beautiful boys at Nuevo Rokoko in Maspalomas, and the superstars at Balans No 34 in Soho (RIP). Thank you for your warmth, shelter and very strong coffee.

About the Author

Dr Paul Taylor-Pitt is an organization development specialist, LGBTQ+ activist, mentor, researcher and coach with 30 years of professional experience in helping people, organizations and systems reinvent themselves. He holds a doctorate in Organization Development Professional Practice, a master's in HR Leadership and an honours degree in Psychology. He belongs to the Society of Authors and is a fellow of the Royal Society of Arts. He has won numerous awards for his work and been featured on several industry lists including People Management's Social Media Power List and *HR Magazine*'s Most Influential Thinkers List. He has created and hosted three podcasts: *HOPECAST, Exploring the Heart of Change* and *Still Here! Still Queer! Now What? The Podcast!* Paul has never had any fun hobbies and worries he is too boring. He lives in London with his husband Dan and their plants, the Sharons. He still misses their cat, Robbie (RIP).

RAISING READERS

Books Build Bright Futures

Dear Reader,

We'd love your attention for one more page to tell you about the crisis in children's reading, and what we can all do.

Studies have shown that reading for fun is the **single biggest predictor of a child's future life chances** – more than family circumstance, parents' educational background or income. It improves academic results, mental health, wealth, communication skills, ambition and happiness.[1]

The number of children reading for fun is in rapid decline. Young people have a lot of competition for their time. In 2024, 1 in 10 children and young people in the UK aged 5 to 18 did not own a single book at home.[2]

Hachette works extensively with schools, libraries and literacy charities, but here are some ways we can all raise more readers:

- Reading to children for just 10 minutes a day makes a difference
- Don't give up if children aren't regular readers – there will be books for them!
- Visit bookshops and libraries to get recommendations
- Encourage them to listen to audiobooks
- Support school libraries
- Give books as gifts

There's a lot more information about how to encourage children to read on our website: **www.RaisingReaders.co.uk**

Thank you for reading.

hachette UK

1 OECD, '21st-Century Readers: Developing Literacy Skills in a Digital World', 2021, https://www.oecd.org/en/publications/21st-century-readers_a83d84cb-en.html

2 National Literacy Trust, 'Book Ownership in 2024', November 2024, https://literacytrust.org.uk/research-services/research-reports/book-ownership-in-2024